CHAKRA HEALING WITH SHADOW WORK

SELF-CARE TO INTEGRATE YOUR SHADOW, UNBLOCK YOUR CHAKRAS, AND BECOME WHOLE

DELPHINA WOODS

HENTOPAN
PUBLISHING

CONTENTS

Introduction 9

1. THE SHADOW 15
   Carl Jung 16
   What Happens When You Reject the
   Shadow 22
   Why You Should Heal and Integrate Your
   Shadow 26
   Shadow Work 27
   Guided Shadow Work Meditation 31

2. THE CHAKRAS 33
   History of the Chakras 34
   Overview of the Seven Chakras 35
   Common Signs Your Chakras Are Out of
   Harmony 41
   Methods for Healing Your Chakras 43
   Chakras and the Shadow 46
   Visualization to Clear Your Chakras 47

3. THE ROOT CHAKRA (MULADHARA) 51
   Themes of the Root Chakra 52
   Common Reasons the Root Chakra
   Becomes Blocked 54
   Signs of an Imbalanced Root Chakra 57
   The Root Chakra and the Shadow 59
   Healing Methods and Tools to Unblock
   Your Root Chakra 61
   Visualization Meditation 70

4. THE SACRAL CHAKRA
(SVADHISTHANA) 73
Lessons and Themes of the Sacral Chakra 74
Common Reasons the Sacral Chakra
Becomes Blocked 76
Signs of an Imbalanced Sacral Chakra 78
The Sacral Chakra and the Shadow 80
Healing Methods and Tools to Unblock
Your Sacral Chakra 84
Visualization Meditation 92

5. THE SOLAR PLEXUS CHAKRA
(MANIPURA) 95
Lessons and Themes of the Solar Plexus
Chakra 96
Common Reasons the Solar Plexus
Chakra Becomes Blocked 98
Signs of an Imbalanced Solar Plexus
Chakra 101
The Solar Plexus Chakra and the Shadow 103
Healing Methods and Tools to Unblock
Your Solar Plexus Chakra 105
Exercises for Healing the Solar Plexus
Chakra 108
Visualization Meditation 114

6. THE HEART CHAKRA (ANAHATA) 117
Lessons and Themes of the Heart Chakra 118
Common Reasons the Heart Chakra
Becomes Blocked 121
Signs of an Imbalanced Heart Chakra 124
The Heart Chakra and the Shadow 126
Healing Methods and Tools to Unblock
Your Heart Chakra 129
Exercises for Healing the Heart Chakra 132
Visualization Meditation 136

7. THE THROAT CHAKRA (VISHUDDHA)   139

Lessons and Themes of the Throat
Chakra   140

Common Reasons the Throat Chakra
Becomes Blocked   142

Signs of an Imbalanced Throat Chakra   145

The Throat Chakra and the Shadow   147

Healing Methods and Tools to Unblock
Your Throat Chakra   150

Exercises for Healing the Throat Chakra   153

Visualization Meditation   159

8. THE THIRD EYE CHAKRA (AJNA)   161

Lessons and Themes of the Third Eye
Chakra   162

Common Reasons the Third Eye Chakra
Becomes Blocked   165

Signs of an Imbalanced Third Eye Chakra   168

The Third Eye Chakra and the Shadow   170

Healing Methods and Tools to Unblock
Your Third Eye Chakra   174

Exercises for Healing the Third Eye
Chakra   178

Visualization Meditation   184

9. THE CROWN CHAKRA (SAHASRARA)   187

Lessons and Themes of the Crown
Chakra   188

Common Reasons the Crown Chakra
Becomes Blocked   190

Signs of an Imbalanced Crown Chakra   192

The Crown Chakra and the Shadow   194

Healing Tools to Unblock Your Crown
Chakra   198

Exercises for Healing the Crown Chakra   203

Visualization Meditation   208

10. INTEGRATION 211
   Common Factors That Negatively Affect
   All Chakras 212
   Exercises for General Healing and
   Integration 215
   Yoga Routines That Help All Chakras 219
   Visualizations and Meditations 226

   Conclusion 231

A Special Offer

From Hentopan Publishing

Get this additional book from Delphina Woods just for joining the Hentopan Launch Squad.

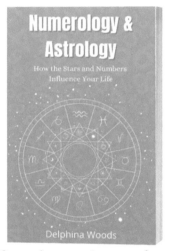

Get your free electronic copy by scanning the QR code below with your phone.

INTRODUCTION

I have a passion for helping people feel whole and healed, so long before my spiritual practice, I trained as a mental health counselor and psychologist. This is where I learned all about Jungian psychology, which has been the core of my career and spiritual path ever since.

Of all the psychological theories I learned about during my education, the most profound concepts were from Carl Jung. He was unique compared to other psychologists, because he took a more spiritual and holistic approach to psychology than his contemporaries. For this reason, he has remained one of the most impactful (as well as controversial) psychologists of the past century.

One of the core concepts Jung developed was the idea of the Shadow self. The Shadow consists of our repressed memories, limiting beliefs, and negative aspects of our psyche to which we are typically blind. According to Jung, many people do not want to see this side of themselves, so they repress them into the Shadow, trying to hide these undesirable elements forever. However, these negative aspects always appear in some shape, particularly in the form of denial and projection.

I had long wondered why so many people (including myself) were blind to their own shortcomings and had a habit of projecting them or denying them altogether. Even clients and peers who were fairly self-aware seemed to have particular blind spots. Jung's concept of the Shadow finally provided an answer to this puzzle. In my opinion, no other psychological concept or theory could explain this phenomenon, especially with the same compassion and understanding.

But this was not the only life-changing concept that Jung introduced me to. His interest in spiritual matters led to his development of important concepts, such as the collective unconscious, dream analysis, and synchronicity. While studying these theories and their implications, I inevitably found myself more and more drawn to the world of spirituality and metaphysics.

Like many other spiritual seekers, I quickly came across the idea of chakras. I was immediately drawn to the concept of the energy body and the fact that much of our lives is governed by our energy flow. Naturally, I was eager to start chakra healing and incorporate these ideas into my sessions with my clients.

While most of the chakra books I read focused on the positive aspects of the chakras, I began to notice a pattern around this topic that few authors addressed. I observed that limiting beliefs and negative thought patterns were a significant reason chakras become blocked in the first place and that working on those beliefs was the key to healthy energy flow. But most people rarely address their limiting beliefs, instead choosing to further repress or hide them. Unfortunately, this only worsens blockages in the chakras, as we can never truly hide or run from these core unconscious beliefs.

After that revelation, it didn't take long for me to connect this idea to the concept of the Shadow. Both are highly influenced by our thoughts and the willingness to heal and integrate our whole selves. Any denial or resistance to healing causes both the Shadow and chakras to suffer. I also realized that healing one helps the other. By working on energy blockages in the chakras, one learns more about and heals their Shadow.

And by doing shadow work, one begins to heal the chakras associated with their particular shortcomings and beliefs.

So while both chakra healing and shadow work are powerful healing tools by themselves, I realized that integrating them can make for a more holistic and powerful healing journey. That's why I wrote this book to be more than a chakra book. It integrates concepts of the Shadow and guides you on how to use shadow work to heal your chakras. By starting this work, you are putting yourself on a path that not only leads to better energy flow but a more peaceful and happily integrated psyche.

The beginning of this book reviews the basics of the Shadow and chakras. If you aren't familiar with these ideas yet, then the first two chapters will help you become familiar enough with them to start your healing work. After that, the rest of the book is dedicated to delving deeper into each of the seven chakras and how they pertain to the Shadow. You will learn what aspects of the Shadow manifest in each chakra and how to heal their particular blockages.

I hope this book can serve as a powerful guide to you during your healing journey. Shadow work and chakra healing are some of the most important healing techniques you will ever experience. Thank you for trusting me to be a part of this life-changing process. Now, let's get to work.

1

THE SHADOW

Let's face it, we all have aspects of ourselves that we don't particularly like. For example, perhaps as a child you were teased for being a chatterbox, so as an adult you restrain yourself from taking part in conversations. Or maybe you feel uncomfortable with your anger, so you repress your emotions. Though we may want to hide our shortcomings and flaws, they are a part of who we are, and hiding them does not make them go away.

Many people also experience negative beliefs about themselves that limit their potential and lives. Much like in the chatterbox example, someone in this situation is limiting themself from having a full social life because they are hiding their true self from the world.

The traits that people are blind to or don't wish to see in themselves are what make up the Shadow Self. Most people repress or reject their Shadow, as confronting their shortcomings or limiting beliefs is often uncomfortable. Unfortunately, no matter how much one rejects their Shadow, it never goes away. Many find that no matter what they do, their Shadow shows up in other areas of their life, or their denial leads to adverse consequences like mental illness or physical disease.

The truth is, it's absolutely essential that your Shadow is healed and integrated in order to feel whole, healthy, and complete. In this chapter, I'll explore the concept of the Shadow—where it comes from, how it affects our lives, and how you can balance, heal, and integrate it to experience complete self-acceptance.

CARL JUNG

The Shadow is a concept that comes from Jungian psychology (which I studied before pursuing a more spiritual path), so we can't discuss the concept of the Shadow without mentioning Carl Jung.

Carl Jung was an early 20th-century Swiss psychiatrist and the founder of psychoanalytic psychology. He was initially a student of Sigmund Freud, but the two eventually went their separate ways due to disagreements in their philosophies. At one point, Freud believed Jung would be his heir and successor to his newly established International Psychoanalytical Association. However, Jung was on his way to developing ideas that would revolutionize both the field of psychology and the realm of metaphysics.

Much like Freud, Jung was very interested in the unconscious mind. While Freud believed that the unconscious was simply a reservoir for repressed memories, urges, feelings, and instincts, Jung had a more positive perspective. He believed that the unconscious was also a source of creativity and healing, and served as more than just a reservoir of survival instincts. But what really made Jung stand out was his idea of the collective unconscious, a concept that I will explain in greater detail below.

Jung eventually broke away from Freud and founded his own school of psychology. Jung was much more spiritual than his colleagues and significantly influenced the popular ideas we see in metaphysics today. Some of his achievements in psychology and metaphysics include:

- Distinguishing between introverted and extroverted personality types

- Understanding the importance of dreams and dream interpretation/analysis
- An emphasis on spirituality and its importance in maintaining good emotional health
- Understanding that two seemingly unrelated events that occur close to one another could have meaning or significance (i.e., synchronicities)

Carl Jung is still a bit of a controversial figure. Many are critical of the spiritual nature of his work, as few psychologists before or since have chosen to integrate spirituality and psychology. Nevertheless, he is considered an important figure and influential psychologist.

Though Carl Jung proposed many influential ideas in the realms of metaphysics and psychology, in order to understand the Shadow, we need to discuss two specific theories of his: the collective unconscious and archetypes.

Collective Unconscious

One of Jung's most revolutionary ideas is the belief in a collective unconscious. Jung believed that all humans share a collection of knowledge and imagery that arises from ancient ancestral experiences. Though humans are unaware of these experiences, this knowledge and imagery are tapped into during times of survival and moments of creativity.

According to Jung, the collective unconscious is why many cultures have similar ideas, beliefs, and symbols despite being vastly different in every other way. This theory also explains why people worldwide have similar fears, such as a fear of snakes or spiders. In art, literature, and symbols, the collective unconscious shows itself in the form of archetypes.

Archetypes

Archetypes are images and themes that come up time and time again in art, literature, symbols, and even in personalities. Almost every culture and time period has at least a few of these archetypes, and you are probably quite familiar with some of them, even if you don't realize it. Jung believed the reason these archetypes show up consistently is because they are pulled from the knowledge and imagery stored in the collective unconscious.

Jung identified a large number of archetypes but paid special attention to four, which he labeled the **Self, the Persona, the Shadow, and the Anima/Animus.** The archetypes exist in our personal lives as well. We may take on one (or more) archetypes as part of our personality, depending on our genetics, background, and experiences.

For example, if your archetype is the Hero, then you will be willing to defy the odds and perform courageous acts to prove your worth. If your archetype is the Sage, you will be more interested than the average person in seeking truth and knowledge. For many people, understanding their archetypes brings about greater self-acceptance and understanding of who they are.

Though all of these archetypes have great importance and influence the lives of millions, one of the most impactful archetypes in both psychology and spirituality is the Shadow.

The Shadow

Simply put, the Shadow is the blind spot of our psyche. It comprises our undesirable traits that we wish to remain hidden from ourselves and other people. Unfortunately, most people are either unaware of or do not wish to confront the darker and unpleasant aspects of themselves, so they don't. This results in the strengthening and dissociation of the Shadow, which causes inner conflict and a feeling of being incomplete.

The Shadow forms when we suppress beliefs, ideas, actions, or anything else that conflicts with those of society or our own values and morals. For most people, this begins in childhood, when we are told how to behave in order to function well in society. Though this is important to learn as a child, sometimes we are led to believe that any unfavorable emotions or actions should be repressed or hidden. As a result, instead of integrating beliefs and emotions in a healthy way into our personality, we suppress them, which creates our Shadow.

When the Shadow forms, so does another archetype: the Persona. The Persona is the mask that we show the world, and is a compilation of the favorable qualities, beliefs, and emotions we are not afraid of or embarrassed about. But it can also comprise fake qualities we take on to present a particular image to others.

Because the Persona is usually perceived as favorably by others, this encourages people to, either unconsciously or consciously, continue rejecting their Shadow and to accept only their Persona. This is a painful process because it means they are rejecting part of who they are.

Many people reject their Shadow because they fear seeing their flaws or what others may perceive as their flaws. For many, the pain of confronting their shortcomings is far worse than rejection, so they continue to ignore their Shadow. However, this can have some severe consequences that affect every aspect of one's life.

WHAT HAPPENS WHEN YOU REJECT THE SHADOW

Many people believe that by rejecting their Shadow selves, they are making their lives better. They think they are successfully hiding their flaws and are showing their true, complete selves. They also think they are successfully hiding negative thoughts and limiting beliefs that could cause distress in their lives and negatively affect their well-being. But no one can completely hide their Shadow. It always finds a way to make itself known, as it is eager to be healed and integrated into our life. Below are the most common ways that the Shadow manifests itself in our lives.

Projection and Denial

Jung stated that when the Shadow is ignored or unknown to a person, it is most likely to be projected. This is the most common way the Shadow shows itself, but few people are self-aware enough to realize it. When people are uncomfortable about a particular trait of their own, they look for that quality in others and project their insecurities onto those people. This temporarily makes them feel better about their own flaws and deflects any responsibility for inner growth.

Of course, rejecting the Shadow can also lead to denial. In many cases, Shadow rejection is unconscious, meaning people are not aware of their undesirable traits or flaws. When confronted, they may deny they have the flaw because they honestly believe it isn't an issue. For example, a person with extreme anger issues may be in denial of their problem. When confronted with the issue, however tactfully, they may fly into a rage and claim they aren't very emotional at all. They may even judge others for showing any emotion, even if it's only a fraction of what they exhibit on a daily basis.

Mental Illness

Rejecting your Shadow can lead to inner disconnect and emotional turmoil. Many people with strong, unintegrated Shadows struggle with negative self-talk, rumination, and low self-esteem. This is incredibly painful to live with and can destroy a person's mental health. If this goes on long enough, it could develop into a mental health condition, such as anxiety or depression.

Other people react to their Shadows in the opposite way. Instead of believing the negative self-talk, they combat it with extreme confidence. This can result in the development of a behavioral disorder like Narcissistic Personality Disorder or Histrionic Personality Disorder.

Regardless of whether someone is struggling with depression or narcissism, both options are unhealthy and avoid the important process of accepting them for who they are.

Dreams

Jung believed that repressed Shadows often manifest in dreams. Since the Shadow cannot get your attention in your waking life, it will communicate with you while you are asleep. For many, the Shadow is represented by dark or ominous figures, such as certain types of animals, monsters, or simply a shadowy presence.

How you interact with this presence can shed light on how you view your Shadow. For example, if you try to interact with the figure, then perhaps you are in the process of integrating your Shadow and are on the path of healing. But if you run away, it could be a sign that you are still avoiding your Shadow and rejecting your true self.

Vices

In order to avoid the pain of the Shadow, some people look to vices to quiet the inner critic and darkness. Habits like smoking, drinking, overeating, and substance use can all temporarily numb the pain. However, these habits do not heal the pain and can actually make it worse. You may have noticed that few people who partake in these habits show any genuine joy or feelings of wholeness.

Harmful Behavior

In some cases, extreme projection can lead to harmful or problematic behavior. That's because sometimes people with strong Shadows mistake others as the source of their pain and perceive them as a threat. For example, sometimes those who are insecure about their sexuality or bodies will exhibit sexist, homophobic, or body-shaming behavior in order to make themselves feel better. They put down people who are secure with themselves because they see them as a threat to their happiness. But as we all know by now, this behavior can have dire consequences. What's worse is that people who are in denial of their harmful behavior will continue to act this way because they need to hurt others in order to feel good about themselves.

Physical Ailments and Illnesses

As many of us already know, many diseases and ailments have their roots in spiritual problems and energy imbalances. Many of the conditions that plague society develop from the tensions and inner turmoil we feel as we try to live in this chaotic world. Much of that tension is caused by the Shadow and our reluctance to heal it.

For example, trauma survivors who hold onto painful emotions often report physical problems, such as fatigue, cardiovascular disease, diabetes, and arthritis. Furthermore, those who reject their anger may develop chronic issues like body aches and pains, as well as high blood pressure. Though you should always talk with your doctor about your physical symptoms, if you are experiencing painful physical ailments, you may find some relief by doing shadow work.

WHY YOU SHOULD HEAL AND INTEGRATE YOUR SHADOW

As we have learned, life is painful, chaotic, and confusing when you reject your Shadow Self. This is why so many people feel incomplete or unsatisfied, but instead of looking inward for healing, they spread their pain to others or find ways to numb it.

The main consequence of rejecting your Shadow is the loss and rejection of your true Self. You cannot be your true Self with only bits and pieces of your personality. You must love every part of who you are and find ways to integrate your shortcomings and limiting beliefs so they can become a positive part of your life. This is why we must all heal and integrate our Shadows; It is the only way we can feel whole and complete.

Many people believe that inner peace comes from always being happy and forcing oneself to feel joyful. This is why many (including authors of popular spiritual books and 'gurus') emphasize forcing yourself to maintain a happy mindset. They truly believe that finding peace is simply a mater of being our "best self" and ignoring the aspects of our personality that we don't like.

But you will never feel genuinely happy until you love every part of yourself. Integration is essential if you want to feel happier, more at peace, and complete.

SHADOW WORK

The practice of healing one's Shadow is called shadow work. It comes in many forms to help you become aware of and accept your flaws and shortcomings. This work incorporates anything that helps you integrate the darker sides of your personality with the lighter ones. It helps you to become whole.

There are many ways that shadow work can benefit your life, including:

- Reduced depression and anxiety
- Increased optimism
- Increased self-love and self-esteem
- More confidence
- Greater creativity
- Stronger connections with others
- Improved clarity

So what does shadow work entail? Shadow work is any activity that helps you explore your inner dialogue, connect with your soul, and encourages self-love. There are many ways to do shadow work. A few options include:

- Journaling (either on blank pages or with prompts)
- Mindfulness
- Meditation
- Recording and analyzing dreams
- Using affirmations
- Working with a therapist

Exercises for Shadow Work

At this point, you are probably eager to get started with shadow work but don't know where to begin. To get you started on your journey, I've compiled some journal prompts and a guided meditation, but before engaging in shadow work, there are a few essential things to understand.

First of all, shadow work is not a substitute for professional guidance from a mental health professional or doctor. If you are struggling emotionally, you may want to consider working with a therapist. This is especially important for trauma survivors who are doing shadow work, as the exercises may bring back memories and cause flashbacks.

It's also important to engage in self-care and self-love during your healing journey. Unlike some other spiritual practices, shadow work brings up raw emotions and deep pain. It is essential work to feel whole and complete, but the process is not easy. You will be forced to look at your flaws and limiting beliefs, which can be challenging for people with low self-esteem. Make sure to go easy on yourself and practice self-love and self-care as much as possible.

Journal Prompts for Shadow Work

Below is a list of journal prompts to help you start connecting with and healing your Shadow. Write as much or as little as you want in response to these questions. Remember, no one has to know what you write, so you're free to respond in any way that suits you best.

- What traits or behaviors in others irritate me and make me judgmental?
- How do I think people perceive me? Is this perception accurate?
- List out your core values. Are you in alignment with them?
- What do I wish people understood about me?
- What things trigger me the most? Why do they bother me?
- Think about someone who hurt you in the past. How do you view them now?
- How do I act when under great stress?
- What is the worst thing I have ever done? What was my motivation for doing it? Were there consequences? Would I still do it today?
- What makes me feel trapped? What does freedom look like to me?
- What in my life gives me purpose?
- What has the most control over my life? Is this healthy?

- Describe yourself with objectivity. Is this difficult?
- What frightens me the most?
- What misconceptions do people have about me?
- What memories bring me shame? What was going on with me during that time, and how have I changed since then?
- What emotions bring out the worst in me?
- What do I dislike most about myself? What can I do to love or improve this part of myself?
- What is the biggest lie I tell myself?

GUIDED SHADOW WORK MEDITATION

Find a quiet place where you can relax and either sit or lie down in a comfortable position. When you are ready, begin to breathe in and out, slowly and deeply. Continue to do this until you feel totally and completely relaxed.

Now, imagine you're in a peaceful field. Maybe you are surrounded by tall grasses or by thousands of lilies. Whatever your field looks like, it brings you a sense of great peace and relaxation.

As you relax in your field, a figure approaches you. Take note of the figure's appearance. Is it a shadowy figure? Is it an animal? Does it look fearsome and angry? Or sad and emotional? This is your Shadow, and it wishes to talk to you. It slowly approaches and sits down next to you.

Now, imagine that your Shadow begins conversing with you. What is it saying? Does it feel abandoned? Is it angry? Is it jealous and critical?

Listen carefully to everything it says. Take note of any memories or pain you feel as it speaks. Is there a certain person or memory that you are thinking about? Do you feel tension in a certain part of your body as your Shadow speaks? Note everything you are feeling and experiencing. If you feel any tension, continue to breathe deeply and slowly to return to the state of relaxation.

When calm again, show compassion and warmth to your Shadow as it speaks to you. Your Shadow wants to be heard and has been through many challenges and trials. It needs your love and acceptance. Give it that by responding compassionately.

Once your conversation is over, hug your Shadow and tell it how much you love and appreciate it. You can also invite it to another session if you like, and repeat this meditation. Make sure it feels welcome to converse with you again. Notice the lightness you feel by doing this.

When you're finished and ready, slowly open your eyes.

2

THE CHAKRAS

Everything is made of energy, including all of us. In addition to our physical body, we have an energetic one. Your energetic body is shaped and manifested by your thoughts, emotions, and movements. Blockages will weaken it, but clearing those blockages will heal it.

The most common way that people tap into their energy body is through chakras. Chakras are wheels of energy that assimilate and express life force energy. Each chakra takes charge of the energy that fuels certain parts of your life and governs specific body parts and essential organs. Though you may not realize it, chakras (and their imbalances) could be responsible for your health, mental well-being, and success or failure in particular areas of your life (such as career or relationships).

When you don't take action to integrate your Shadow, these energy wheels can become blocked, which can have devastating consequences for your health, well-being, and other parts of your life. In this chapter, I'll explore in detail the concept of chakras and explain why shadow work is so crucial to healing them.

HISTORY OF THE CHAKRAS

Though chakras may seem like a fairly novel New Age topic, the fact is that chakras have been around for a long time.

The concept of chakras is thousands of years old and was first documented in the early texts of the ancient traditions of Hinduism. Chakras were initially mentioned in the Vedas and Upanishads (written in the second and first millennium BCE, respectively). However, they were much simpler and different from the way we envision chakras today. Later on, chakras appeared in medieval Buddhist texts and became more prominent in medieval Hindu texts. The Buddhist chakra system typically only had four or five chakras, while ancient and medieval Hindu systems included six or seven. Since the seven-chakra system is the most well-known, this is the one I will focus on in this book.

Chakras were introduced to Western culture in the late 1800s, and much of the lore we know about them today was added at this time. For example, it was Westerners (specifically the color system of Charles W. Leadbeater's 1927 book *The Chakras*) who gave the chakras a rainbow color scheme, and it wasn't until the past few decades that chakras were associated with tarot, astrology, witchcraft, and other spiritual topics. There were quite a few prominent Western thinkers and spiritualists who expanded our understanding of chakras. Today, most of what we know about chakras is quite different from what you may read about them in ancient Hindu or Buddhist texts.

Even though chakras have been in Western culture for nearly 150 years, it is only in the past 50 years or so that they have become a mainstream topic. Now, almost everyone in Western culture understands their importance or at least knows about how chakras affect our health and well-being.

OVERVIEW OF THE SEVEN CHAKRAS

As I said, the most popular chakra system is the seven-chakra system introduced in ancient Hinduism. The seven chakras (from bottom to top) in this system are:

- Root (Muladhara)
- Sacral (Svadhisthana)
- Solar Plexus (Manipura)
- Heart (Anahata)
- Throat (Vishuddha)
- Third Eye (Ajna)
- Crown (Sahasrara)

Each chakra in the system is located somewhere along the spine and governs the life energy associated with a particular area of your health and life. Below is an overview of each of these seven chakras, but we'll go into more detail about each one in upcoming chapters.

Root Chakra

Also known as the Muladhara (which translates to "root" and "base"), the root chakra is located at the base of the spine, right near the tailbone area. It is an important chakra that helps with grounding and connecting to the earth. People with a blocked or unbalanced root chakra are often ungrounded and feel they don't have the right to take up space. It is the chakra of safety and security, which are essential before focusing on and healing other areas of one's life.

The root chakra is also connected to issues involving the bladder, colon, and lower back. Some people even associate this chakra with issues regarding the feet or legs. Muladhara is symbolized by the color red and is associated with the element of Earth.

Sacral Chakra

The sacral chakra is located just above the root chakra, right below the navel area. Also known as Svadhisthana (which means "where your being is established"), this chakra is in charge of the energy we use for creativity, sexuality, and sensuality. So when you're struggling with your artistic endeavors or intimacy with your partner, this is probably the chakra you need to clear and heal. The sacral chakra is also considered the storehouse for most emotions, so many emotional and mental health concerns are connected to this chakra.

The sacral chakra governs all issues related to the sex organs, hips, and kidneys. It is represented by the color orange and is associated with the element of water.

Solar Plexus Chakra

Above the sacral chakra, you'll find the solar plexus or Manipura (which translates to "lustrous gem") in the upper navel and stomach area. The solar plexus is the chakra of confidence and assertiveness. A robust solar plexus helps a person develop good self-esteem and use their power and will to achieve their goals and dreams. Conversely, a weak solar plexus makes a person passive and weak-willed.

The solar plexus also plays an essential role in regulating the stomach, kidneys, liver, and adrenal glands. It's also a part of the sympathetic nervous system and is usually the chakra that is blocked when you are struggling with anxiety. This chakra is represented by the color yellow and is associated with the element of fire.

Heart Chakra

Though no chakra is more important than any other, the heart chakra tends to get more attention than the others. Also known as Anahata (which roughly translates to "unbeaten"), the heart chakra governs all matters of the heart. From self-love to relationships to compassion and forgiveness, this chakra stores all the energy associated with anything that can pain or heal your heart. An open heart chakra allows us to connect fully with others and exhibit unconditional love, while a closed chakra can lead to loneliness, anger, distrust, and insecurity.

As you may have guessed, the heart chakra is located in the center of the chest and is in charge of the lungs, heart, and breasts. It is the center chakra in the seven-chakra system and, therefore, also represents the balance of spiritual and earthly matters. It is represented by the color green and is associated with the element of air.

Throat Chakra

The first of the upper chakras is the throat chakra, also known as Vishuddha (which means "purest"). The throat chakra is located at the base of the throat and governs all matters of communication, such as public speaking and the ability to speak your truth. When this chakra is blocked, you may be more timid and unwilling (or unable) to speak your mind. When balanced, you can communicate clearly and assertively.

As you can probably guess, this chakra governs all matters of the throat and is connected to issues such as sore throats and laryngitis. It is also connected to any problems involving the thyroid and mouth. This chakra is represented by the color blue and is associated with the element of sound.

Third Eye Chakra

The third eye chakra (also known as Ajna, which means "perceive") is another chakra that garners a lot of attention and discussion. That's because it's seen as a more spiritual chakra than the ones already mentioned. Located at the brow (just above and between your other eyes), the third eye chakra is associated with all matters relating to intuition, dreams, and spiritual gifts (such as clairvoyance and telepathy). It also helps with concentration and focus and is your gateway to communicating with Spirit. A blocked or unbalanced third eye will prevent you from connecting with the Universe or your intuition, while an open third eye will help you with these and will help you access your spiritual gifts.

The third eye chakra is connected to all issues involving the pineal gland. It is represented by the color indigo and is associated with the element of light.

Crown Chakra

The final chakra in this system is the crown chakra, also known as Sahasrara (which translates to "thousand petals"). The crown chakra is your connection to Spirit. It is the gateway to the rest of the Universe and is the chakra you use to communicate with God. If this is blocked, you will have difficulty hearing your divine guidance and communicating with Spirit. You may also struggle to feel one with the Universe and will feel very disconnected. This chakra also is associated with all matters regarding consciousness, thought, and intellect.

Unlike the other chakras, the crown chakra, as the name suggests, is not located directly on the body but right above the top of the head. It is represented by the color violet (or sometimes white) and governs the element of thought.

COMMON SIGNS YOUR CHAKRAS ARE OUT OF HARMONY

When your chakras are out of harmony, so is your life. The life force in each chakra controls the flow of energy in certain areas of your life, as well as the health of particular body parts. Therefore, when your chakras are blocked or unbalanced, you will experience poor mental health, physical ailments, and problems with your finances, career, relationships, and more.

Poor Mental Health

Whether energy is stuck and stagnant or active and chaotic, the energetic change will certainly affect your mind. As a result, you may experience too much energy, which makes you anxious or too little energy, which encourages negative thoughts and melancholy. Many people with blocked chakras live with mental health conditions like anxiety, depression, obsessive-compulsive disorder, and ADHD, but find healing and balance once they begin to heal their chakras.

Some mental health conditions are tied to a specific chakra, which makes healing much more straightforward. Other conditions are more complex and may require healing multiple chakras before you experience any relief. However, if you are experiencing any mental health conditions, you should also work with a mental health professional, as they will know the best treatment strategy for your situation.

Physical Ailments

Each chakra governs organs, essential systems, and body parts that we need to function healthily on this planet. Therefore, if any of your chakras are out of balance or harmony, you may experience body pains and diseases. For example, having a blocked heart chakra may result in heart disease, while a blocked sacral chakra can make one impotent or cause a UTI. Some severe cases of blocked chakras may lead to chronic conditions or even organ failure.

Though chakras can influence your physical health and contribute to various ailments, it is always crucial to talk to a medical professional about other factors, as well as treatment options. Though doing shadow work and energy healing is important, a medical professional will help with the physical healing.

Life Challenges

In addition to health concerns, chakras maintain and control the energy that flows into other areas of your life. Your finances, career, and relationships are all governed by chakras, so if any of them are blocked, you will experience stagnant energy in that particular area of your life.

For example, if you have a blocked or weakened root chakra (the chakra of safety and security), you may struggle to make enough money to pay your bills. If you have a blocked or weakened throat chakra, you may struggle to assert boundaries and be clear about your needs. If you have a blocked crown chakra, you may feel completely disconnected from your spiritual life.

When faced with problems in life, we must take action to tackle them head-on. However, by doing shadow work and healing our chakras, we can encourage better energy flow that will increase our chances of success.

METHODS FOR HEALING YOUR CHAKRAS

Though it can be overwhelming to see just how much the chakras affect every aspect of your life, luckily, thousands of years of knowledge are at your fingertips. Over the centuries, spiritual seekers have found many methods to heal the chakras and bring one's soul and life back into harmony. Though I'll provide specific exercises in later chapters, here are a few general tips for healing your chakras.

Yoga

Nothing helps the energy flow like yoga. Just like the chakras, yoga is an ancient concept that originated in India. Over the centuries, the practice has been altered and refined to help as many people as possible create a healthy energy balance and flow.

There are multiple forms of yoga and thousands of poses to choose from. Many of those are specifically designed to help with energy blockages in and around the chakras. I'll provide some poses and sequences to try out when I discuss each chakra in more detail.

Meditation

Meditation clears and settles the mind, allowing one's energy to calm and heal. Though meditation is always beneficial, it is a particularly effective practice when healing energy and doing shadow work. Most people utilize guided meditations or affirmations during meditation, but even simple mindfulness meditation can be incredibly healing.

Visualization

Visualization is a powerful tool to help you manifest your dreams as well as heal your energy and body. We are powerful creators, so what we visualize often becomes reality. Therefore, when dealing with stuck and stagnant energy, visualizing healthy energy flow can help unblock your chakras. If you want to try this yourself, I've included a general visualization for chakra healing at the end of this chapter.

Journaling

Journaling is particularly effective for energy healing, especially when combined with shadow work. Journaling allows you a safe space to write down all your thoughts, releasing blocked energy as you do so. In a world that isn't always compassionate, a journal can be a great friend to help you work through your limiting beliefs and past traumas that keep your energy stagnant.

Self-Care

Our physical and energetic bodies are intertwined; an injury to one affects the other. Therefore, simply taking care of yourself can do wonders for your chakras.

One way to do this is by following a healthy, nutritious diet. Each chakra is associated with particular food and food groups that can help heal it. For example, when balancing the root chakra, eating red foods as well as earthy foods that are grounding can be helpful.

Exercise is another great way to keep energy flowing and keep chakras unblocked. Whether going for a run, swimming, or simply taking a stroll through nature, moving your body will get the energy flowing.

CHAKRAS AND THE SHADOW

The primary reason chakras become or remain out of harmony is due to our unconscious beliefs. For example, if you believe you aren't deserving of love, then you probably will have a blockage in your heart chakra. That energy will remain stagnant until you work on this belief and feel worthy of receiving love from others.

Unhelpful unconscious beliefs, like the example above, and the repressed parts of ourselves form not only our Shadow but also the blockages in the chakras. Chakras only remain balanced and open when we fully accept and love ourselves. This means knowing, understanding, and healing the darker sides of ourselves that we are uncomfortable with. Therefore, shadow work and integration are absolutely critical, as no one can fully accept themselves and be open if they have not healed and integrated their Shadow.

So how do you go about integrating shadow work and chakra healing? There are a couple of ways to do this. First, you can do shadow work to identify your flaws, unconscious beliefs, and other shortcomings and use this discovery to identify which chakras are blocked. Or, if you can easily identify which chakras are blocked, use this knowledge to learn more about your Shadow.

In the following chapters, I will discuss in detail how the Shadow shows up in each chakra and how to identify which specific chakras are blocked. I'll also provide exercises to help you with each chakra's shadow work and chakra healing. For now, I will end this chapter with a visualization to help start clearing all your chakras and energy body.

VISUALIZATION TO CLEAR YOUR CHAKRAS

Now that you have a general overview of the chakras, it's time to start working on balancing them. Though later chapters will provide specific exercises on how to heal each individual chakra, here I've provided a visualization that will go through each one and begin the healing process.

Find a quiet area for your visualization and sit or lie down in a comfortable position. Begin by breathing deeply and slowly to get into a relaxed state.

Now visualize a bright red center at the bottom of your spine. Feel the warmth and energy in that area of your body. This is your root chakra, also known as Muladhara. Imagine it swirling freely and glowing brightly. Let this energy ground you to the Earth and protect you. Feel free to speak some affirmations such as "I am grounded" or "I am safe."

Next, move on to your navel, where the sacral chakra, or Svadhisthana, lies. Visualize the beautiful shade of orange and how it illuminates your whole navel area. Imagine it flowing freely without blockages or stagnation. Do you feel your sexual energy coming alive? Or perhaps your creative energy? Take some time to breathe through any emotions you feel or to speak affirmations such as "I am creative" or "I am sensual."

Repeat this process for the other five chakras. Visualize the solar plexus at the top of your stomach, your heart chakra in your chest, your throat chakra in your throat, your third eye on your brow, and the crown chakra on top of your head. Imagine their bright color and their flowing energy. Continue to breathe deeply as all that stagnant energy is released. Feel free to repeat any affirmations that come to mind during the process.

Once you have gone through each chakra, continue to breathe deeply. Visualize all seven chakras now, all spinning brightly. Notice how good your energy feels. Take a few minutes to enjoy this and get in tune with your energy body. When you are ready, take a few deep breaths and then slowly open your eyes.

3

THE ROOT CHAKRA
(MULADHARA)

Color: Red
Organs: Bladder, Colon, Feet, Legs
Location: Bottom of the spine; tailbone
Element: Earth
Mantra: Lam
Planet: Mars
Animals: Elephant, Mole, Ox, Hippo, Skunk

All healing begins at the roots.

Though other healers may disagree, I personally believe that the root chakra is the most important. Why? The root chakra is our literal foundation on this planet. It roots us to the Earth and provides the energetic support we need to build a fulfilling life.

Without a healthy root chakra, it will be far more difficult to heal your other chakras or conduct successful shadow work. We can't build a happy life or have a successful healing journey without a foundation, and the root chakra is that foundation.

Therefore, it is essential that this chakra is balanced and healed before working on the others. Without further ado, let's explore the importance of the root chakra, how it relates to the Shadow, and how you can heal it to create an energetic foundation and feel safe.

THEMES OF THE ROOT CHAKRA

The root chakra does not get enough love, but as the foundation of our life, its energy influences much of our lives. Everything you need to create a stable and healthy foundation for life is connected to your root chakra. Let's break down all the important themes that come up with this chakra.

Security and Survival: The first important theme of the root chakra is survival. A healthy and balanced root chakra helps us obtain everything we need to survive, including food and drink, shelter, and money. These are the absolute bare minimum requirements to survive on this planet and create a foundation for better things. A healthy root chakra helps us acquire these things with ease; an imbalanced root chakra makes survival much harder.

Safety: It's not enough to survive on this planet; we need to feel safe. The root chakra helps us to create a safe environment and to leave any situation that isn't good for us. When this chakra is imbalanced, it can be much harder to feel safe or take action to become safe. Furthermore, an imbalance can block or disrupt the fight or flight response and even attract situations that put us in danger.

Grounding: We need to be grounded to stay in the present and overcome our challenges. Even with security and safety, life has a way of manifesting situations that can temporarily uproot us. A healthy root chakra grounds us and provides us with solid roots into the earth. This allows us to stand firm, even when situations shake us up. But without solid roots, we can easily be uprooted and struggle to navigate life's difficulties. An imbalance can also make it harder to focus on goals and dreams and instead make us feel ungrounded, directionless, and spacey.

The Right to Exist: If we feel like we don't belong on this planet, then it will be much harder to acquire all that we need to survive. People who feel unworthy to exist have a much harder time having their basic needs met and achieving their dreams. Nothing else can be achieved if we don't believe we deserve to exist in the first place.

COMMON REASONS THE ROOT CHAKRA BECOMES BLOCKED

Though life can be difficult with any blocked chakra, a blocked root chakra makes life particularly challenging. Without a solid foundation, you will struggle to build the life of your dreams. Very little healing can be accomplished if you don't feel safe and secure in the world in the first place. This is why I believe spiritual seekers should focus on healing their root chakras first.

But how does this chakra become blocked in the first place? Unfortunately, due to the nature of the root chakra and the areas it governs, it becomes blocked by traumatic events that make us feel unsafe or insecure in the world. Below are a few common reasons people experience blocked chakras.

Abuse: Abuse, especially early in life, can make someone feel like they are unworthy of love and don't deserve to exist. Abuse not only puts someone in a perpetual state of fear and danger, but it is often partnered with manipulation and other tactics that make the victim feel unworthy of happiness. Abuse is a complex situation that affects multiple chakras. Still, first and foremost, it hinders a person from creating a good foundation in life or even believing that they deserve that foundation at all.

Neglect and Abandonment: Likewise, neglect and abandonment can also create a sense of not belonging or deserving to belong. When someone neglects you (especially a parent or loved one), it can feel as though the whole world is rejecting you or telling you that you don't deserve the things you need to survive. It can be very hard to overcome that thinking, especially if this neglect happened at a young age and its source was someone who was supposed to care for you.

Accidents, Surgeries, Injuries: Experiencing a horrible accident, injury, or terrible side-effect of a surgery can traumatize the body into thinking it is not safe. Depending on the nature of the incident, it can alter the mind and body for a lifetime, making it much harder to heal. It can be difficult to feel safe and grounded again, because we worry that the incident will happen again or we believe our life will never be complete or fulfilling as a result of it.

Poor Boundaries: In some cases, traumatic issues or events occur due to poor boundaries. Poor boundaries allow neglectful or hurtful people into your life and tell the world that your needs don't matter. This allows these people to rule over your life and neglect or abuse you as they see fit.

Inherited Trauma: If you know you're experiencing severe issues with your root chakra, but none of the above situations apply to you, then it is possible that you inherited trauma from your parents or previous generations. When our parents or grandparents experience significant trauma without healing, it can affect their behavior and thinking for the rest of their life. It's easy for children to absorb fear and anxiety without realizing it or understanding where these emotions came from. Therefore, even if you had a healthy and stable childhood, it's possible that you have absorbed and inherited some trauma. This is common for descendants of refugees or survivors of war or genocide.

Because of the seriousness of the issues that cause imbalances in the root chakra, I always recommend working with a mental health professional when working on root chakra healing. Healing this chakra may cause flashbacks, raise bad memories, and spark nightmares, and it can be overwhelming to heal from these past events. A mental health professional can help you work through your past safely and keep you grounded as these memories and emotions arise.

SIGNS OF AN IMBALANCED ROOT CHAKRA

Since the root chakra is essential to survival and safety, it can cause significant problems in every area of your life when imbalanced. Without a healthy root chakra, it can be extremely likely experience mental health concerns, physical ailments, and/or significant imbalances in your life. Below are some of the most common issues of an imbalanced root chakra.

Common mental health and emotional concerns stemming from an imbalanced root chakra:

- Persistent fear or anxiety
- Feeling ungrounded and spacey
- Feeling disconnected from your body
- Feeling disconnected from Earth or believing you don't belong here
- Believing that you are unworthy to exist or take up space
- Body dysmorphia
- Post-traumatic stress disorder (PTSD)
- Depression
- Panic attacks
- Suicidal thoughts**

If you are experiencing suicidal thoughts, it's important to talk to a mental health professional.

Common physical ailments and diseases that occur from an imbalanced root chakra:

- Eating disorders
- Issues with the legs and feet
- Problems with the bladder and colon (such as constipation or a UTI)
- Lower back problems
- Feeling sluggish, lethargic, and fatigued
- Prostate problems
- Knee pain
- Sciatica

Common life challenges due to an imbalanced root chakra:

- Struggling to find a safe home or dealing with homelessness
- Developing an unhealthy focus on spirituality that encourages you to neglect your basic needs and responsibilities
- Struggling with essential self-care, such as basic hygiene, staying hydrated, and eating a balanced diet
- Financial problems (such as not making enough money to pay bills)

- Spending more time dreaming than taking action
- Feeling like you don't belong anywhere
- Being stubborn and afraid of change

THE ROOT CHAKRA AND THE SHADOW

When it comes to the root chakra, it's pretty clear how well it connects to the concept of the Shadow. For many people, trauma is the main reason they become disconnected from parts of themselves and develop limiting beliefs that rule their lives. As a result, many live solely by their negative thoughts and often repress certain aspects of their personalities into their Shadows in order to feel safe.

The root chakra is also the chakra of fear, which happens to be the governing emotion of the Shadow. If we are deeply afraid of life or were abused and neglected, we will repress our fears, limiting beliefs, and self-worth into the Shadow in order to hide our fear. But as we know now, the Shadow does not stay hidden. Instead, it appears in various areas of our lives, most commonly as projection. It also shows up in our actions and habits, even if we are in denial.

For example, a child living in a low-income family may grow up extremely frugal, even if she makes a decent living as an adult. Her traumatic experiences of not having enough as a child may make her hoard her wealth instead of spending it on things that could improve her life. While she may have more than enough to create a great life for herself, she refuses to do so out of fear of losing her financial security in the future. She may not realize she is doing this because she has repressed her financial and security fears to her unconscious Shadow.

Another prime example is someone who has experienced abuse. The experience may have made them feel that they are unworthy of love and have no right to exist. These beliefs are often pushed into the unconscious Shadow, so abuse survivors are unaware of them. However, they may self-sabotage their happiness and well-being (e.g., by entering into another abusive situation or not tending to their health).

Therefore, the Shadow qualities that usually come up with the root chakra are fears that the person in question will be unsafe in the future (i.e., will repeat past traumas) or that they do not deserve safety or to happily exist in the first place.

HEALING METHODS AND TOOLS TO UNBLOCK YOUR ROOT CHAKRA

Though the root chakra may contain some difficult memories and limiting beliefs to overcome, there are many ways to help with the healing process. Everything from changing your habits to incorporating your spiritual tools can help bring more balance to your life and strengthen your foundation. Below are a few methods and tools to try out if your root chakra is out of harmony.

Crystal Healing

Working with crystals is a great way to help balance and unblock your energy. Crystals contain healing energies and vibrations that can clear out blockages and bring your energy back into balance. There are hundreds of crystals found all around the globe, and many of them are associated with specific chakras.

When looking for a crystal to heal the root chakra, you want something that will help ground you and protect you as you heal from your past. These crystals should also help you build a strong foundation as you unblock any negative energy from your root chakra. Some crystals that can help out with this are:

- **Garnet:** A gorgeous red gem that provides life, energy, and support when you feel drained. Helps revitalize you after years of hardship and pain.
- **Red Jasper:** A comforting red stone that helps you build and strengthen your foundation and keeps you rooted and grounded.
- **Black Tourmaline:** A powerful stone of protection that absorbs and protects you from harmful and darker energies.
- **Bloodstone:** A beautiful stone that keeps you connected to the earth and grounded in your power.
- **Black Obsidian:** Another protective stone that shields you from harmful energies.

Essential Oils

Essential oils can help calm your emotions and can keep you grounded while you work on your healing. They also can help bring forward the positive gifts and lessons of each chakra and balance the shadow aspects. To utilize essential oils, you can use them in a diffuser, put a few drops in a bath, or apply them to your skin. If you choose the latter, make sure to dilute them with a carrier oil and do a patch test to ensure you won't have an adverse reaction.

For the root chakra, you want to choose essential oils that are earthy and will ground you. Therefore, choose oils from trees and earthy-smelling plants to bring your energy back to the earth. A few great options to choose from include:

- Cedarwood
- Frankincense
- Patchouli
- Vetiver
- Sandalwood

Diet

Another great way to balance your root chakra is by eating root-chakra-balancing foods. This includes foods that will help you ground yourself or are the same bright hue of red as this important chakra. Some foods that can help heal your root chakra include:

- Strawberries
- Tomatoes
- Raspberries
- Cherries
- Red apples
- Red peppers
- Beets

- Root vegetables (potatoes, carrots, turnips, onions)
- Ginger
- Turmeric

Exercise

Exercise is another effective way to ground yourself and help you reconnect with your body. When you exercise, you have to pay attention to what your body is doing if you want to realize the most beneficial results. Exercise can also make you strong, which will help you feel safer as you navigate this scary world. Though most exercises can help with these issues, here are a few options that I recommend:

- Martial arts/Self defense
- Running
- Swimming
- Walking in nature

Exercises for Healing the Root Chakra

In addition to the tools mentioned above, below are some shadow work exercises and a few other tips that will help you unblock your root chakra and integrate this part of your Shadow.

Journal Prompts

Journaling is essential for healing past traumas and working through limiting beliefs. Though many people do well with journaling on blank pages, sometimes prompts can help you focus on the particular issues you wish to heal. Here are a few prompts that will help you on your journey to healing the root chakra and your past traumas.

- When life feels chaotic, what can I do to feel grounded and centered?
- What does it mean to be rooted in the present moment?
- How can I cultivate the feeling of being grounded and present in my life?
- What can I do to ensure I feel safe despite external circumstances?
- What are some of the most beautiful memories I have?
- Who or what reminds me that I'm physically safe?
- Complete the sentence: "I have felt unsupported when..."
- What am I ready to let go of?
- What can I do to better support myself?

- When I think about my basic needs (food, shelter, money), how do I feel? Do I feel safe and secure or afraid and worried?

Affirmations

Affirmations help rewire our brains to break through limiting beliefs and replace them with positive ones. Below are some affirmations that will open your root chakra, encourage your body to feel safe, and help you believe that you deserve to exist on this beautiful planet.

1. I am safe and secure.
2. I am grounded.
3. I belong.
4. I am prosperous and abundant.
5. I have everything I need to survive and thrive.
6. I am strong.
7. I am strongly rooted to the Earth.
8. I am connected and grounded.
9. I deserve to take up space.
10. I deserve to be safe at all times.
11. I am worthy of respect.
12. The Universe will always provide.
13. All is well in my world.
14. I am supported by Mother Earth.
15. I am safe in my body.

16. I have a strong foundation for my life.
17. I have a right to be here.
18. I am rooted in this present moment.
19. I am connected to my body.
20. I trust in the good of the world.

Yoga Poses

Yoga is an essential exercise for anyone who needs to unblock energy. For the root chakra, you should focus on poses that connect you to the earth, provide support, and strengthen you. I've compiled some of my favorite poses that I use to keep my root chakra clear.

Balasana (Child's Pose): Sit on your heels and lean forward, resting your head on the ground. Rest your arms beside your legs, palms out. For a greater stretch in the hips, move your legs further apart. You can also extend your arms out in front of you. This is a great pose to get support from the earth and surrender.

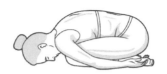

Sukhasana (Easy Pose): This is a simple sitting pose. Cross your legs into a comfortable sitting position and enjoy grounding into the earth.

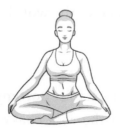

Malasana (Squat Pose): From a standing position, slowly move down into a squat, ensuring your tailbone is close to the ground. Keep your heels on the floor to stay rooted.

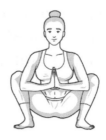

Tadasana (Mountain Pose): Stand straight and tall and plant your feet firmly into the ground to fully root yourself.

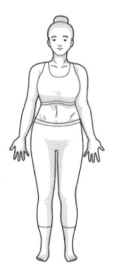

Virabhadrasana (Warrior II): Keep both feet firmly planted on the ground. The front foot should face forward while the other faces the side. Extend the front leg into a lunge and lift your arms out to the sides for a powerful, strengthening stance.

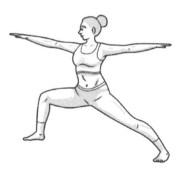

Savasana (Corpse Pose): Simply lie down comfortably with your arms at your sides and palms wide open. Feel safe, knowing that the earth fully supports you in this pose.

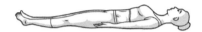

VISUALIZATION MEDITATION

Find a comfortable spot in which to sit or lie down. To begin grounding yourself, breath calmly, deeply, and slowly. Feel your breath bringing you back into your body. Wiggle your toes and be present to all the sensations you can feel throughout your body. Notice all the tension and emotions calming down with every breath you take. Keep breathing deeply until you feel serene and centered in your body.

Now, imagine a red light glowing at the end of your tailbone. Notice what a brilliant shade of red it is and how it feels. Take note of the warm and grounding feeling in the lower half of your body. This light is your root chakra, and it is rooting you to the earth. It is keeping you grounded and safe.

As you breathe in and out, allow this light to get bigger until it encompasses your whole body. Notice that it is creating a shield around you, protecting you from all harm. Allow yourself to relax and feel safe as this light shields you.

Allow this light to protect you for as long as you need. Continue breathing during the process to keep you grounded and present during this experience. If you wish, you can say a mantra or affirmation such as "I am safe" or "I am grounded." Or you can repeat the syllable "Lam." Do whatever you feel guided to do as this loving red energy strengthens and protects you.

When you are ready, allow the energy to condense again to your tailbone. Know that it will always be available to protect you and keep you safe. Thank your root chakra for protecting you. When you are finished, take a few more breaths and slowly open your eyes.

4

THE SACRAL CHAKRA (SVADHISTHANA)

Color: Orange
Organs: Sex Organs, Hips, Kidneys
Location: Navel/Lower Abdomen
Element: Water
Mantra: Vam
Planet: Moon
Animals: Dolphin, Frog, Crocodile, Otter, Fish

Life is at its fullest when we are creating and expressing ourselves.

After forming a solid foundation with the root chakra, we move into the emotional realm of the sacral chakra (also known as Svadhisthana). Where the root chakra helps us to feel that we have the right to exist, a healthy sacral chakra establishes our right to feel and experience life. Once survival issues have been attended to, it is time to enjoy life by creating and enjoying pleasurable activities.

But when the sacral chakra is blocked, it is much harder to experience joy and pleasure. We feel shame for having emotions, are blocked from our creativity, and are prevented from having one of the most enjoyable experiences of humanity: sex.

Life is more than just working, eating, and sleeping. It is full of art and pleasure and experience. So let's explore how the sacral chakra helps us with these things and how to unblock it to fully enjoy this life we are given.

LESSONS AND THEMES OF THE SACRAL CHAKRA

The sacral chakra governs the core aspects that allow us to enjoy life. Without any enjoyment, life is just a game of survival or a large to-do list. Let's break down all the core themes that come up with this chakra and how it teaches us to make the most of our lives.

Pleasure: Without pleasure, it is difficult to find any satisfaction in life. Pleasure allows us to feel joy and pursue any activity that gives us a much-needed break from our work. The sacral chakra helps us experience pleasure and creates or attracts opportunities that give us more of this feeling.

Creativity: All humans have a passion to create. Whether it be an artistic endeavor or building a business, we all create something at some point in our lives. Creation and using our creativity are core to what makes us human. The sacral chakra is the storehouse of creative energy and helps us to express this energy in a way that is unique to us.

Sexuality: The epitome of pleasure and creation is the act of sex. It is one of the most enjoyable activities humans can experience and produces the ultimate creation: that of life. A healthy sacral chakra is essential for a safe and satisfying sex life. A blocked chakra will result in too little sex, and an excessive chakra may lead one to engage in unsafe sexual activity.

Desire: We cannot build a great life without desiring it first. People with blocked sacral chakras often find they have little desire for anything and therefore don't manifest anything good. An unblocked sacral chakra helps us attune to our inner desires so that we can manifest them into the physical world.

Flexibility, Flow, and Surrender: The sacral chakra helps us to be flexible to our surroundings and situations, so we can always enjoy the present moment no matter what is happening around us. It also helps us surrender to Divine Will and stop micromanaging the Universe. When this chakra is blocked, it can result in rigid and inflexible thinking, which makes it much harder to find joy in the moment.

Emotions: Life is only enjoyable because we can experience positive emotions and compare them to negative ones. Without these emotions, we would all be like Spock from Star Trek or a computer. Though many emotions can be influenced by other chakras, the sacral chakra is the primary center that allows us to experience and regulate our emotional experiences.

COMMON REASONS THE SACRAL CHAKRA BECOMES BLOCKED

Since the sacral chakra is the core of our emotional lives, quite a few situations can cause it to become blocked. Below are the most common situations, but anything that harms your feelings about sex or creativity, or adversely impacts your emotions will negatively affect this chakra.

Adverse Experiences: Any adverse event that is highly emotional to experience can cause an imbalance of emotions and an energetic blockage. This can include but is not limited to grief, divorce (or your parents' divorce as a child), or abuse. Undergoing such a negative situation and not having the proper coping mechanisms can lead to a habit of either repressing emotions or becoming overly emotional.

Sexual Abuse: For some, a fear of or negative perspective on sex is linked to previous sexual abuse. Sexual abuse is a traumatic and terrifying ordeal that violates our safety and boundaries. It ruins something that is natural and beautiful. It's important to note that though the sacral chakra is the central sex chakra, sexual abuse often affects multiple chakras and takes significant work to heal. I recommend working with a therapist in addition to utilizing other healing methods and tools.

Sexual Shame: Many people also have blocked sacral chakras because they feel shame around sex. This can be due to parallel issues of feeling unworthy of love or intimacy, or can be caused by absorbing the dominating views on sex expressed by authority figures, such as parents, or society. Sex is a highly complex issue that society struggles to navigate. It is only in recent years that information about sex has been communicated more openly, with healthy sex tips being the priority. However, there are generations of people who were subjected to unhealthy beliefs about sex, which can make it hard for them to have fulfilling sexual experiences.

Denial of Pleasure or Creativity: Many people (whether the result of their upbringing, a toxic work culture or something else) unconsciously deny any enjoyment, pleasure, or creativity in their lives. Modern culture often views these facets of life as things that get in the way of success. But pleasure makes life worth living and is a primary reason why we work hard every day. A person with a blocked sacral chakra will deny themselves this enjoyment and live to work rather than work to live.

Denial or Shaming of Emotions: Many people believe that supressing their emotions makes them go away. However, in my experience, this only leads to disease and suffering, as that energy has to manifest in some form. We evolved with emotions, whether we like them or not, so we can't just numb them or run away from them. Denying your emotional needs will only cause more pain and result in a severely blocked sacral chakra.

SIGNS OF AN IMBALANCED SACRAL CHAKRA

Since the sacral chakra primarily governs emotions, pleasure, sex, and creativity, these are the areas of life that will be significantly affected if this chakra is blocked. Below are the mental health concerns, physical ailments, and life challenges that arise from a blocked sacral chakra.

Common emotional and mental health concerns that arise from a blocked sacral chakra include:

- Extreme emotions and turbulent mood swings
- Problems with emotional regulation
- Obsessive attachment/attachment disorders
- Lack of excitement or passion for life
- Fear of sex/low libido
- Denial of pleasure and fun
- Emotional disconnect
- Loneliness
- Fear of change
- Addiction

Common physical ailments that develop from a blocked sacral chakra include:

- Lower back pain
- Sexual problems
- Hip issues
- Anemia
- Ovarian cysts
- Issues with the spleen and kidneys

- Fatigue and low energy
- Painful premenstrual symptoms or premenstrual dysphoric disorder (PMDD)

Life challenges that manifest from a blocked sacral chakra include:

- Either a poor sex life or an overactive and unsafe sex life
- Struggles with creativity, such as writer's block
- Difficulty manifesting goals and dreams
- Poor social skills/struggling to socialize with others
- Poor boundaries that toxic people take advantage of
- Rigid and stubborn thinking
- Inability to "go with the flow"
- Life overall is dreary and unenjoyable

THE SACRAL CHAKRA AND THE SHADOW

In the sacral chakra, the Shadow takes the form of shame. When people feel insecure about their creativity, emotions, or sexual life, they project their insecurity onto others by shaming them from enjoying these same aspects of life. This is because they also feel shame for wanting to enjoy life, so they project that shame and perpetuate the cycle. Let's look deeper into why they do this.

Shaming of Artists and Creators: When it comes to creativity, the Shadow most commonly shows up in how we view artistic careers. This has become a more prominent issue in recent years, given increased opportunities for people to engage in and monetize creative endeavors. Because this is such a new trend, many people (primarily from older generations) may not consider these opportunities as real professions and will often instruct creative people to "get a real job."

The truth is that these people are carrying a deep inner resentment against these younger professionals for pursuing their passions. These careers are often much more fun and satisfying than the more traditional careers of decades past. People who resent others for choosing these careers often wish they'd had such opportunities when they were younger. But instead of making any positive changes in their own career, they resent those who take the leap. They project this resentment as judgment and shame, and pressure artists to "get a real job" so they will be miserable just like them.

Shaming and Denial of Emotions: Another common way the Shadow shows up in the sacral chakra is the denial, shaming, and judgment of emotions. Many people (particularly men) are raised to believe that emotions make a person seem weak, so they should never feel or express them. As a result, they deny their emotional needs and judge others harshly who express their feelings.

However, though they usually aren't aware, their emotions project in many other ways. For example, most of us have had that boss who is always irate and yelling at employees. At the same time, he denies he is an emotional person and has little awareness of his feelings. Emotions can also manifest in mental illness or even a physical disease. Many studies are beginning to show the link between emotions and illness, with countless people dying every year because they denied their emotional needs. That's why this particular Shadow issue is a grave concern that needs more attention and awareness.

Shaming of Sex: Of course, I can't end this section without discussing how the Shadow affects our views and judgments on sex. As we just discussed, these days more and more people are openly communicating about sex and enjoying healthier and more satisfying sex lives. However, many people grew up with unhealthy or limiting sexual perspectives or were restricted from sex due to cultural or religious beliefs, so it's common to see the Shadow arise in judgment against sexually free people. People who are insecure in their own sex lives and sexuality, in general, will judge and persecute those who do not have these limiting views.

Major social issues arise from people who do not heal this particular Shadow issue. For example, millions of women have recently lost abortion and sexual health rights, and people of all sexualities and genders are persecuted daily because of who they desire to have sex with. Since the powers that be have very limited views on what sex should be and who should enjoy it, they feel threatened by all those who enjoy it in ways that don't align with their limited views. This is an excellent example of how ignoring your Shadow can have significant consequences.

If you experience shame in any of these areas or you shame others for these issues, then these are major concerns you need to heal. Shame is a powerful emotion that prevents us from loving life and becoming a unique individual (which is the theme of the next chakra). Shame literally prevents you from moving forward into your consciousness. Therefore, if you can't heal the shame surrounding the core aspects of the sacral chakra, it will be much harder for you to strengthen your will and self-esteem when healing the solar plexus chakra.

HEALING METHODS AND TOOLS TO UNBLOCK YOUR SACRAL CHAKRA

Since the sacral chakra is in charge of so much, you can probably find numerous opportunities for healing. When looking to heal the core facets of the sacral chakra, you'll find many healing tools that can help you with this process. Below are some crystals, essential oils, and foods that will help you with your healing journey.

Crystals

When looking for crystals for the sacral chakra, you want to find something that boosts creativity, enhances sexual energy, and helps you process emotions. There are quite a few options that meet these criteria, including the following:

- **Carnelian:** An orangish or reddish-brown stone that boosts libido, helps heal sexual issues and inspires creativity.
- **Orange Calcite:** A bright orange crystal that heals negative emotions in the body and enhances creative gifts and talents.
- **Citrine:** A yellowish stone that helps balance emotions and activates creativity.

- **Sunstone:** An orangish stone that heals negative emotions.
- **Tiger's Eye:** A tiger-striped stone that helps heal depression, anxiety, and other strong negative emotions. It also helps balance mood swings and encourages a calmer, more rational mindset.
- **Moonstone:** A whitish stone that helps calm and heals turbulent emotions.
- **Amber:** A crystal made of fossilized tree sap that helps absorb negative emotions and energies and balances the mind.

Essential Oils

To heal the sacral chakra, you need essential oils that help calm and balance emotions and encourage joy, pleasure, creativity, and flexibility. A few oils that can bring about these positive emotions include:

- Ylang ylang
- Rose
- Sweet orange
- Tangerine
- Patchouli
- Helichrysum
- Sandalwood
- Neroli

- Jasmine

Diet

The best foods to heal your sacral chakra include anything that exhibits the same bright orange color as the chakra itself. Luckily, there are many delicious foods that show off this vibrant color. A few of them are:

- Carrots
- Mangos
- Apricots
- Sweet potatoes
- Oranges
- Orange peppers
- Nectarines
- Butternut squash

In addition to these foods, you should also make sure to consume moist foods or food with lots of water. This includes fruit with high water content, soup, or even smoothies. The element of the sacral chakra is water, so you need to ensure your body is properly hydrated!

Exercises for Healing the Sacral Chakra

In addition to the tools mentioned, I've also provided some shadow work exercises and a few other tips that will help you unblock your sacral chakra and integrate this part of your Shadow. However, healing the sacral chakra can be an emotional process, so make sure to take it easy and give yourself plenty of self-care.

Journal Prompts

When journaling for the sacral chakra, you want to get to the roots of why you may not be enjoying life as much as you would like. Are you experiencing any emotional concerns? Blocks in your creativity? Is your sex life unfulfilling? Below are a few journal prompts to get you started.

- What can I do to find more opportunities for play?
- What are ten things I love about my body?
- Where can I be more energetic and creative in my life?
- How do I treat people in my life? Do I give them space? Do I have healthy boundaries?
- What is my view on sex? What influenced this?
- I feel most creative when...
- How can I bring more joy into my life?
- What can I do to regulate my emotions when they feel overwhelming?
- Five hobbies I would love to explore include...
- How can I manifest my desires better?

Affirmations

Affirming your birthright to feel pleasure, desire, creativity, and sexuality is a great way to start healing your sacral chakra. Below are some affirmations that will rewire you to believe that you deserve to feel and enjoy life.

- I deserve to feel pleasure.
- Life is pleasurable.
- I embrace and celebrate my sexuality.
- I deserve to enjoy life.
- I accept the flow of life.
- I express my emotions in a healthy way.
- My creativity flows effortlessly.
- I am an empowered sexual being.
- I have the power to manifest my dream life.
- My sexuality is sacred.
- I am clear with my boundaries.
- My body is sacred to me.
- I give myself permission to prioritize pleasure and creativity.
- I honor my emotions.
- I am healing my emotions.
- I am connected to my creative energy.
- Abundance and passion for life are flowing through me.
- Joy is my birthright.

- My life is full of joy and creativity.
- I feel safe enjoying sex.

Yoga Poses

Since the sacral chakra is located in the lower stomach, the best yoga poses are those that utilize that area and help open the hips. Below are a few yoga poses that help with this.

Dvipada Pitham (Bridge Pose): Lie down on your back, bend your knees (so they are pointing towards the sky), lift up your hips, and tuck in your chin. You can keep your arms parallel to your body or interlace them underneath your hips.

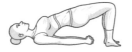

Jathara Parivrtti (Abdominal Twist Pose): This is a simple pose that provides numerous healing benefits. Simply lie down, then twist your hips and legs to the side with the legs stacked up on each other.

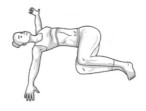

Kapotasana (King Pigeon Pose): Only do this pose if you are very flexible or have practiced yoga for a very long time. From a kneeling position, lean your head and shoulders all the way back and curve backward until your head touches your feet. Keep your hips raised to open them up so they get the most healing.

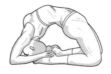

Supta Baddha Konasana (Reclining Bound Angle Pose): Lie down, bringing your knees up and letting your legs gently fall to either side so they face outward, forming a diamond shape. Place one hand on your stomach and the other on your heart.

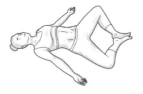

Mandukasana (Frog Pose): Begin on all fours in a tabletop position. Slowly widen the distance between the knees without overextending yourself. Next, bring the arms down to the floor and keep your elbows at shoulder distance.

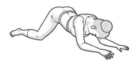

Utkata Konasana (Goddess Pose): Begin in a standing position and move your feet a few feet apart. Point the toes away from each other and do a slight squat. Raise your arms and bend the elbows at a 90-degree angle.

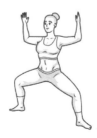

VISUALIZATION MEDITATION

Find a comfortable spot to sit or lie down. Begin to breathe deeply to keep yourself centered and grounded. The sacral chakra is the storehouse of emotions, so opening it may result in an emotional release. If this happens, don't fight your emotions, but continue to breathe deeply to keep yourself grounded during the experience.

As you breathe deeper and deeper, notice how much calmer you're becoming. Notice any tension or emotions within you. Note their presence and where you feel them (such as in your knees, your chest, your hips, etc.), and keep breathing through the tension. Breath until you feel serene.

Now, bring your attention to an orange light glowing at your navel. It is a vibrant shade of orange that exhibits joy and radiance. Imagine this orange wheel of light spinning happily. This is your sacral chakra, and it is healing your painful emotions and providing you with the energy needed to enjoy life. As your sacral chakra keeps spinning, you may feel some tension in your lower stomach. This is your chakra unblocking all the tense energy that has been preventing you from feeling joy. It is normal and will pass soon. Just keep breathing.

Once you feel your chakra unblocking, imagine the orange light filling your entire aura. Feel the happiness, joy, and freedom that comes with such a radiant light. Notice how you feel lighter, as though the burdens of the world are off your shoulders. It's time to have some fun and enjoy life a bit more. Let this light fill you with the joy that you deserve.

Stay in the orange aura for as long as you need. If you've been overworked lately or don't allow yourself to be happy often, then you may need a long soak in this orange light. During this time, you can repeat some mantras to further the healing process, such as "I deserve to be happy," "Life is pleasurable," or "I embrace my creativity." Whatever affirmations pop into your head that promote happiness, sexuality, or creativity are encouraged.

When you are ready, allow the energy to condense again to your navel. Know that it will always be available when you need a boost of happiness or creativity again. Thank your sacral chakra for its healing. When you are finished, take a few more breaths and slowly open your eyes.

5

THE SOLAR PLEXUS CHAKRA
(MANIPURA)

Color: Yellow
Organs: Stomach, Kidneys, Liver, Adrenal Glands, Intestines, Pancreas, Spleen
Location: Upper Stomach
Element: Fire
Mantra: Ram
Planet: Sun
Animals: Bear, Ram, Lion, Tiger, Dragon

Once our physical and emotional needs are met, we must carve our own path and tell the world who we are. At this point, we are no longer reactive out of survival nor caught up looking for more pleasure. Now we can focus on using our energy to define who we are and manifest a life that fits our desires. To create a happy and satisfying life, we must have a solid understanding of who we are, have the autonomy to go after what we want, and develop the confidence and inner power needed to achieve our dreams. These are all matters governed by the solar plexus chakra.

When the solar plexus (also known as Manipura) is blocked, we are passive, give our power away to other people, and don't develop a solid identity. When it is plagued by the Shadow, we feel powerless and are threatened by those who honor their inner power. A healthy solar plexus is essential if you want to feel good about who you are and have some control over your life. If you struggle to feel powerful or find yourself manipulated and ruled by others, you need some solar plexus healing. Let's dive into this important chakra and discuss how healing it can empower you.

LESSONS AND THEMES OF THE SOLAR PLEXUS CHAKRA

In general, the solar plexus provides us with the energy to form our full identities. We cannot create a truly satisfying life if we do not even know who we are. Understanding our identity requires confidence, autonomy, inner power, and the vitality to go after our desires. The solar plexus helps with all these characteristics.

Confidence and Self-Esteem: Life is much harder when you lack confidence. A lack of confidence prevents people from applying for the job they want, asking people out on dates, or working towards their goals. It also makes them easier to manipulate. People with low self-esteem rarely take action toward their goals and instead find themselves puppets in other people's lives. A healthy solar plexus is essential for a strong sense of confidence.

Of course, a healthy balance is crucial. Too little confidence causes inertia and passivity, but too much makes us narcissistic and can drive away the things and people we want. A healthy solar plexus allows us to experience an appropriate level of confidence that gives us the energy and inner power to carve our path in life.

Autonomy and Will: One of the most important aspects of human existence is having a sense of autonomy. We all need the independence to be ourselves and forge our own path, even if we have a strong support network or people who will follow us along the way. How often do we let our will be undone and allow others to make decisions for us? For many, the answer is all too often. Developing a healthy sense of autonomy and enacting your will helps create a solid sense of identity and prevents you from being manipulated by others.

Power: Society has a complicated relationship with power because power is often mistaken for authority. Authority figures use their power to put other people down and bend them to their will. But real power is internal and allows us to stand firm against these manipulations. Power is needed to carve out your destiny. Without this inner power, you can easily become passive, complacent, and resentful for allowing others to dim your light.

Energy and Vitality: To have success in the above areas and have the ability to carry out our goals and dreams, we need energy and vitality. Many powerless people are often lethargic, sluggish, and fatigued. That's because they don't have enough energy in their solar plexus to power their will. A blocked solar plexus can't provide you with the energy you need to reach your goals. An open and healthy solar plexus gives you the vitality and energy to tackle all challenges and achieve your destiny.

COMMON REASONS THE SOLAR PLEXUS CHAKRA BECOMES BLOCKED

We live in a culture full of people who love to inflate themselves and tear others down. This, unfortunately, leads to many situations that can block the solar plexus chakra. If you have weak boundaries or are more susceptible to judgment, then it's very likely that at some point, someone has taken advantage of you and has torn down your confidence. From parents and peers to societal expectations, we often encounter people and beliefs that tear down our inner power. Below are some common scenarios in which this can occur.

Pressure to Conform: Though the world has billions of unique individuals, cultures encourage their people to conform to a sense of 'normal.' Though younger generations are learning to resist this pressure, many people still struggle with this and hide their true selves in order to avoid judgment and shame. But when we hide ourselves, we deteriorate our self-esteem and drain our inner power.

Shame: Much like with the sacral chakra, the solar plexus is plagued by the demon of shame. Shaming in any form can shake any person's emotional foundation so they forget to stand in their power and act with will and autonomy. Whether you're shamed for your actions or your outfits, any form of shaming may be affecting the health of your solar plexus chakra.

Strict Parenting: Sometimes parents must be strict to protect their children or teach them important life lessons. However, some parents choose to see their children as extensions of themselves instead of independent individuals. As a result, they control every action and decision the child makes, which destroys the child's sense of autonomy and will. This causes the child to become dependent on their parents and unable to navigate the adult world alone.

Abuse or Punishment from Authority Figures: Unfortunately, parents are not the only ones who believe they have the right to control others. This is a common occurrence in corporate culture, where employees are forced to be loyal. At the same time, their employers remain domineering and take away their free will. Authority figures believe they must abuse or punish their subordinates to keep them in line and get them to do what they want. But this rarely creates the loyalty they seek and instead destroys employees' self-esteem and decision-making skills.

Cultural/Societal Beliefs About Power: Even if someone does not experience the issues above, they may have a blocked solar plexus chakra from absorbing the negative cultural beliefs surrounding authority and power. All over social media, you will see people expressing their anger and helplessness, as they believe they are unable to do anything to counter the evils done by the authorities of the world. It's easy to absorb this message and believe you are helpless and instead become passive. Every person on this planet was put here to fulfill a mission that combats this darkness, but we can't succeed at our mission without inner power.

SIGNS OF AN IMBALANCED SOLAR PLEXUS CHAKRA

When the solar plexus is imbalanced, we are passive, experience inertia, and feel helpless in this world. Though the root chakra is our energetic foundation, it will still be weak without the energy and strength of the solar plexus. Below are the mental health, physical ailments, and life challenges that arise from an imbalanced solar plexus chakra.

Common emotional and mental health concerns that arise from a blocked solar plexus chakra include:

- Low self-esteem
- Passivity
- Aloofness
- Poor self-discipline
- Victim mentality/blaming others
- Agitation/pent-up energy
- Releasing emotions in unhealthy ways, such as through extreme anger and temper tantrums
- Narcissism and selfishness
- Nihilistic mindset

Common physical ailments that develop from a blocked solar plexus chakra include:

- Eating disorders
- Chronic fatigue
- Digestive issues
- Diabetes
- Hypertension
- Hypoglycemia
- Pancreas problems
- Gallbladder issues
- Liver problems
- Addiction

Life challenges that manifest from a blocked solar plexus chakra include:

- Being easily manipulated by others
- Struggling to take action toward goals and dreams
- Having a weak will or being unable to act on it
- A stubborn and rigid attitude
- Struggling to make decisions
- Others take control of your life and your major decisions
- A habit of shaming or judging others to feel better about yourself

- Feeling powerless against and unable to resolve life's challenges

THE SOLAR PLEXUS CHAKRA AND THE SHADOW

The forms that the Shadow takes in the solar plexus are quite familiar to most people. I argue that collectively, the world is working to heal its solar plexus, as many themes of authority and power have come to light in recent years. This is why so many are struggling with feelings of powerlessness, and even authority or selfishness. When we consider many of the major events happening today, we can see these themes playing out time and time again. Let's delve deeper into the ways the Shadow manifests itself in the solar plexus.

Abuse of Authority and Power: The abuse of authority or power is the most common way we see the Shadow of the solar plexus. Governments worldwide are struggling as their citizens gain more freedom and tap into their inner power. Some governments handle these changes well, while others double down on acts of punishment and repression. Governments who respond with threats and by taking away their citizens' free will are acting out of the solar plexus Shadow. They feel threatened when their people decide to live for themselves, and respond with threats and violence to maintain their power.

On a smaller scale, we can see the Shadow arise through this chakra when we see people with a bit of power (such as managers and CEOs) abusing that power to punish others and make them feel small. These people have blocked their solar plexus, and are using their power and salaries to hide the inner shame and low self-worth they feel. Instead of looking within for healing, they take out their pain on subordinates who don't swear complete loyalty or stroke their boss's ego.

Shame: The fact is, any form of shaming can come from the solar plexus Shadow. While shaming related to creativity or sex is often from the Shadow of the sacral chakra, forms of shaming related to self-worth, actions, or individuality come from the Shadow of the solar plexus chakra.

Narcissism: On the flip side, too much confidence can produce a solar plexus Shadow in the form of narcissism. It's commonly believed that narcissists actually have incredibly low self-esteem that they need to hide in order to feel better, and this is why they develop a grandiose sense of self and tear down others. Instead of learning to heal their fragile self-esteem, they need to exaggerate their accomplishments and see others in emotional pain in order to feel good about themselves.

HEALING METHODS AND TOOLS TO UNBLOCK YOUR SOLAR PLEXUS CHAKRA

Improving your confidence, vitality, and inner power is no simple task. You will need to utilize many tools and exercises to help you firmly connect with your true power. Luckily, there are crystals, essential oils, foods, and exercises that can help.

Crystals

When choosing crystals to help you on your journey, you want gemstones that have the same vibrant yellow luster of the solar plexus but also that help you boost your confidence, vitality, and inner power. Below are a few options.

- **Citrine:** A yellowish stone that strengthens one's self-esteem and promotes positive thinking.
- **Amber:** This crystal (made of fossilized tree sap) helps absorb negative emotions and improves confidence and self-esteem.
- **Yellow Jasper:** A yellow-brownish gem that attracts positivity and boosts self-confidence.

- **Calcite:** An orangish stone that flushes negativity and makes room for more self-confidence and positivity.
- **Tiger's Eye:** A tiger-striped stone that encourages and establishes more confidence, self-esteem, and willpower.
- **Yellow Topaz:** A gorgeous, lustrous gem that strengthens faith in yourself and optimism.
- **Lemon Quartz:** A light yellow quartz that helps to build confidence and courage while also improving quick decision-making.
- **Yellow Tourmaline:** This yellow version of tourmaline helps protect you from negative energy while boosting your confidence and courage.
- **Sunstone:** An orangish stone that increases vitality and helps boost independence. It also improves confidence and strengthens boundaries.
- **Carnelian:** A sunset-colored stone that stimulates inner fire, light, and life. It boosts vitality and motivation and activates your inner warrior spirit.

Essential Oils

The best essential oils for the solar plexus chakra are oils that will boost your vitality and renew your sense of optimism. A few options that can help with this include:

- Lemon
- Ylang ylang
- Neroli
- Juniper
- Sandalwood
- Spearmint
- Mandarin
- Geranium
- Chamomile
- Cypress
- Rosemary

Diet

When looking for foods that will help your solar plexus chakra, you want food options that have the same bright yellow vibrancy of this particular energy center, as well as anything that will give you the energy to manifest your destiny. Some options include:

- Bananas
- Lemons
- Corn
- Pineapple
- Yellow squash

- Yellow bell peppers
- Oats
- Brown rice
- Rye
- Beans

Exercise

Just as with the root chakra, exercise is essential for healing the solar plexus. Exercise (especially activities that strengthen the core) gives us the strength and vitality needed to stay healthy and enjoy life. Though any exercise will help unblock the solar plexus, I recommend anything that uses up any excess pent-up energy or strengthens your body and makes you feel more powerful. A few options include:

- Martial arts
- Strength training
- Running
- Swimming
- Dancing

EXERCISES FOR HEALING THE SOLAR PLEXUS CHAKRA

Healing the aspects of your Shadow that are tied to your solar plexus can be particularly challenging. With this chakra, you must come to terms with the fact that you are responsible for your life and must take action to achieve your destiny. These are difficult challenges to overcome, but I've provided some journal prompts, affirmations, yoga poses, and a visualization to help you out.

Journal Prompts

When journaling to heal the Shadow of your solar plexus, it is essential to analyze the themes of self-worth, power, and authority in your life. Your perspective on these topics determines how much you allow yourself to fully live in your life and be yourself. Below are a few prompts to get you started.

- When do I feel most confident? When do I feel least confident? What can I do to develop more confidence?
- What is my relationship to authority?
- How did my upbringing shape my opinion of authority?
- Do I allow myself to feel and express anger? How can I express my anger in a healthy way?
- Do I act according to my own will and goals or those of other people?
- What can I do to act more from my own will and personal power?

- What aspects of myself am I ashamed of? How can I learn to love those aspects more?
- Are there times when I shame others for being different? How can I be more supportive?
- Do I healthily express my individuality, or do I just go with the crowd?
- What does it mean to be empowered? What can I do to empower myself more?

Affirmations

When stating affirmations to heal the solar plexus, it is essential to find affirmations that give you a sense of inner power. You want to strengthen your confidence and identity so you can go out into the world being your full self without any shame. Below are some affirmations that will do just that.

- I honor the power within me.
- I accomplish tasks easily and effortlessly.
- I can do whatever I will myself to do.
- I value myself as I am.
- I am strong, powerful, and confident.
- I am ready to face any challenge.
- I am worthy just as I am.
- I stand in my power.
- I am worthy of love, happiness, and success.
- I am whole and complete.

- There's nothing I need to do or be to earn love or respect.
- I own my power and recognize the strength inside me.
- I can accomplish incredible things.
- I believe in my abilities.
- People value my work, my time, and my skills.
- I confidently and fearlessly believe in myself.
- I am proud of all that I have accomplished.
- I can do anything I set my mind to.
- I can create positive change in my life.
- I hold the key to my own happiness.

Yoga Poses

The best yoga poses for the solar plexus help strengthen the core and promote overall strength, power, and flexibility. These are all essential for achieving your dreams and developing your confidence and inner power. Below are some yoga poses that will help you.

Navasana (Boat Pose): From a sitting position, slowly straighten out your legs and raise them so they are at a 45-degree angle from the floor. Lean your torso and head back so your body is making a V-shape. Reach your arms straight out in front of you so your body looks like an upside-down A. If you struggle with this pose, you can place your hands behind your legs for support.

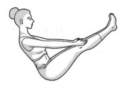

Purvottanasana (Reverse Plank Pose): Sit on the floor, straighten out your legs and place your hands a few inches behind your hips. Bend your knees, flatten your feet on the ground and lift your hips. Your body should take the shape of a scalene triangle.

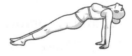

Virabhadrasana II (Warrior II Pose): Keep both feet firmly planted on the ground. The front foot should face forward while the other faces to the side. Extend the front leg into a lunge and lift your arms out front and back for a powerful, strengthening stance.

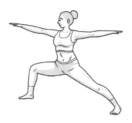

Dhanurasana (Bow Pose): Lie flat on your stomach. Lift your legs behind you and then your head and neck. Grab your feet with your hands to put your entire body into a gentle U-shape.

Anjaneyasana (Low Lunge Pose): From a standing position, move down into a lunge, ending with one leg at a 90-degree angle and the other lying flat on the ground behind your body. Once centered, lift your arms straight up to the sky with your palms facing each other.

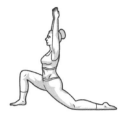

Adho Mukha Svanasana (Downward Facing Dog):
From a standing position, bend forward and place your
hands on the floor. Now walk your legs back so your
body makes a downward V-shape. Relax your head
between your arms or rest it all the way on the ground
if you have the flexibility to do so.

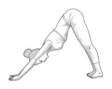

VISUALIZATION MEDITATION

*Find a comfortable spot to sit or lie down. Now take some
slow and deep breaths to release any tension and get yourself
into a calm and serene state.*

*Once relaxed, begin to envision yourself drawing energy
from the earth. This energy enters through your root chakra
and slowly rises through your body. It helps ground you
through the root chakra and balances any emotions or*

tension you feel as it rises through the sacral chakra. After visiting these two chakras, it slowly makes its way to your solar plexus.

As it enters the solar plexus, feel your chakra begin to open up and activate. You may feel some tension or sensations in your upper stomach as this happens. This is normal; just keep breathing through it. Once your solar plexus receives this energy, visualize its bright yellow rays swirling happily in your upper stomach. Witness how bright and vibrant the color of this chakra is. Notice any vitality or happiness you feel when you activate this chakra.

Now allow that yellow color to surround your entire body. Feel how your body is soaking in these yellow rays, building its confidence and feeling more positive by the minute. Feel your inner power strengthening and your determination building. Your solar plexus is helping you to become strong in your power. Feel how powerful you are with this incredible yellow light lifting you up.

Spend as long as you like in these yellow rays. If you've been experiencing low self-esteem or depression recently, you may want to visualize your yellow shield for a while longer. Feel free to speak any affirmations, such as "I am powerful" or "I value myself as I am," to enhance the healing. This is your time to feel powerful and strong, so you can visualize or say anything that helps you experience power and strength.

When you are ready, allow the energy to condense again to your stomach. Know that it will always be available to give you that vitality and confidence boost you may need. Thank your solar plexus for its healing. When you are finished, take a few more breaths and slowly open your eyes.

6

THE HEART CHAKRA (ANAHATA)

Color: Green
Organs: Lungs, Heart, Breasts, Chest, Thymus Glands
Location: Center of Chest
Element: Air
Mantra: Yam
Planet: Venus
Animals: Deer, Antelope, Dove, Lovebird, Wolf, Dog

Once you've begun to tap into your inner power and develop your individuality, it's time to learn how to truly love yourself as you are. The self-discovery that comes with healing the solar plexus leads to discovering some of your deepest flaws and shortcomings. Though working on your confidence and self-esteem can help you to heal and accept these shortcomings, you won't experience true self-acceptance without self-love. Confidence arises from our belief in our strengths; self-love arises when we accept every aspect of ourselves. The heart chakra (also known as Anahata) is the chakra of self-love and, therefore, is the key to self-acceptance.

Though every chakra is important, the heart chakra plays a special role when integrating the Shadow. We can't face our Shadow and heal it without having a strong sense of self-love. We need to look at our blind spots and negative traits with self-acceptance, which cannot occur without loving ourself. We also need to forgive anyone who has hurt us and contributed to the development of our Shadow. The heart chakra governs all aspects of love, including forgiveness and compassion, so healing it is absolutely essential to healing and integrating your Shadow. Now let's explore the role of this vital chakra and how it can be healed.

LESSONS AND THEMES OF THE HEART CHAKRA

Without love in our lives, either for ourselves or for other people, life can be a sad and lonely experience. The heart chakra governs all matters of love and the heart, which includes romantic matters, connections with friends, and our relationship with ourselves, all of which are important to a fulfilled and happy life. Below are the common themes and lessons that the heart chakra teaches us.

Love and Relationships: As you can surmise from its name, all forms of love and all kinds of relationships (partnerships, friendships, connections with family members, etc.) are affected by the heart chakra. A healthy heart chakra helps us maintain these relationships and create boundaries that avoid toxic ones.

Self-Love: The most important relationship is the relationship you have with yourself. You won't have a positive relationship with your soul without self-love. A healthy heart chakra helps to find that balance in which you love yourself as you aren't blind to your shortcomings. This is a critical attribute to master if you wish to fully heal and integrate your Shadow.

Unconditional Love: Many people believe that true love is the kind of love displayed in movies and television shows. It is often very dramatic, with lots of fighting, tension, and sexual activity replacing true connection. But genuine unconditional love is not toxic, shallow, or selfish. Unconditional love is when we love someone despite their flaws or past transgressions. We see the person exactly as they are and choose to love them anyway. We love them no matter what they do, and don't expect anything in return. This doesn't mean that the love has no problems, but they are usually settled in a healthy and respectful manner. Unconditional love is difficult to achieve, but the heart chakra must be fully open to truly love and connect with another human being in this manner.

Trust: We cannot fully connect with anyone if we do not trust them. Sometimes trust is eroded for a valid reason, such as after an affair or some type of betrayal. But we can also be naturally distrusting because of previous experiences or negative societal beliefs (such as all men are cheaters or all women are shallow). The heart chakra teaches us why trust is essential in healthy relationships and gives us the discernment we need to determine who deserves our trust.

Forgiveness: Forgiveness is one of the highest spiritual qualities anyone can attain on the path to enlightenment, but it certainly isn't easy to achieve. When people wrong us, it is easy to hate and judge them forever. But holding onto that hurt doesn't help you or them. The heart chakra helps you change your perspective of the person who wronged you so you can let go of your judgment and forgive them.

Balance: The heart chakra is smack in the middle of the seven-chakra system. It helps to connect the earthly matters of the lower chakras with the more spiritual matters of the upper chakras. As a result, this chakra helps us to balance all these matters, since one side is not more important than the other.

COMMON REASONS THE HEART CHAKRA BECOMES BLOCKED

In a world where people regularly hurt and tear each other down, it's very common for people to have a blocked heart chakra. People who don't love themselves rarely look within for healing and instead hurt others, thinking it will relieve them of their pain. Self-love is a topic that has only recently gained traction in our modern culture, and most people still struggle with it.

Furthermore, though more people today are gaining confidence and self-esteem, there isn't much attention or teachings focused on loving others, so people continue to hurt each other, which only causes more pain. Let's review some common situations that can block a heart chakra.

Grief: Nothing is more heartbreaking than losing a loved one. When a loved one dies or breaks up with us, the loss is excruciating and it's difficult to heal. It takes months or sometimes even years to recover and build a new life. The heart chakra takes the brunt of this pain, blocking and closing itself off to prevent further pain.

However, for some people, the pain lingers for years, leading to a long-lasting blockage.

Abuse: I've mentioned abuse a few times already, but it can't be stated enough how harmful it is to your mental health and energetic system. Abuse shatters our sense of survival, our identity, and our ability to love ourselves and trust other people. When abuse occurs, it's easy to become fearful of others and assume they will hurt you just as your abuser(s) did. The manipulation of an abuser can also convince us that we aren't worthy of love or affection. This is a very common and understandable reason why the heart chakra becomes blocked.

Shame: As you've probably noticed by now, shame is another common theme with chakra blockages. It is a major reason why we struggle to love ourselves. At some point, some person shamed us and made us believe that we were unlovable or unworthy of happiness. Shame teaches us that we should feel bad about who we are, which directly hinders our ability to love ourselves. And yet, shaming is still quite socially acceptable, leading to many blocked heart chakras.

Betrayal: There are few situations more gut-wrenching and heartbreaking than betrayal. Whether it be an affair or discovering a friend lied about something significant, betrayal of all kinds is a dagger to the heart. It can be hard to trust anyone again or believe you will connect with someone who won't betray you. It's understandable that people who have experienced betrayal have a severe blockage in their hearts.

Rejection: It's hard to bounce back when we are rejected by people we care about. Whether being rejected for a first date or being asked for a divorce, rejection is an incredibly painful experience that can easily make a person feel unlovable. Sometimes rejection is ruthless, but even respectful rejections (such as tactfully turning someone down for a date) can still be taken personally and cause a significant heart chakra blockage.

Other Negative Past Experiences with Friends, Family, or Partners: When the people we love treat us poorly or violate our boundaries, it can completely destroy our sense of self-worth. If we allow toxic people into our lives (or can't get away from them), they can erode any self-love or compassion we may have for ourselves. The people we spend the most time with directly influence our mindset, so toxic people or negative experiences with friends and family can cause a heart chakra blockage and significantly reduce self-love and compassion.

SIGNS OF AN IMBALANCED HEART CHAKRA

A lack of self-love can manifest in a myriad of ways. Whether it results in standoffish and aloof behavior or chasing love out of desperation, the symptoms will be unique to the individual. But there are some patterns in mental health symptoms, physical health concerns, and life challenges that tend to manifest from an imbalanced heart chakra.

Common emotional and mental health concerns that arise from a blocked heart chakra include:

- Low self-esteem
- Depression
- Loneliness
- Narcissism
- Fear of intimacy or love
- Aloofness or antisocial behavior
- Lack of empathy
- Shyness
- Anxiety
- Fear of being alone

Common physical ailments that develop from a blocked heart chakra include:

- Heart disease or other heart conditions
- Issues with the lungs
- Immune system deficiency
- Asthma
- Circulation problems
- Bronchitis
- Problems with thymus glands

Life challenges that manifest from a blocked heart chakra include:

- Lack of relationships or a support network
- Unable to connect with others
- Poor boundaries
- Co-dependent and clingy
- Lack of forgiveness
- Lack of empathy and compassion
- Overly judgmental
- Overly defensive
- Jealousy, hatred, and holding grudges
- Not being able to move on from past relationships or connections
- Difficulty trusting people

THE HEART CHAKRA AND THE SHADOW

The Shadow manifests in the heart chakra in ways that destroy our most profound connections with others as well as our connection with ourselves. When the heart chakra is blocked, we experience a meager amount of self-love, so we overcompensate through our interactions with others. Because this is such a common issue, there are quite a few ways the Shadow can manifest.

Grudges and Hatred: One of the most common ways the Shadow arises in the heart chakra is through grudges and feeling hatred toward another human or toward oneself. Hatred can develop in response to someone's unjust behavior or because our low self-esteem was triggered by the person we hate. Hatred is often connected to jealousy and judgment, which arise when a person feels inadequate. When people feel unworthy or inadequate in some way, they often take out their pain by hating and judging someone else rather than healing their own pain.

Twisted Concepts of Love: When people lack love for themselves, they look to others to fill their empty cup. They believe that the emptiness and pain they feel can be healed by having certain friends or being in certain kinds of relationships. Eventually, they get the idea that potential partners exist to serve and heal them instead of seeing them as independent humans to love and cherish. This type of love becomes toxic and possessive and rarely leads to any genuine connection. Unfortunately, few people gain self-awareness of this issue, as television and movies reflect and perpetuate these toxic concepts of love.

Neediness, Anxious Attachment, and Desperation: On a similar note, many people become very needy, dramatic, and overly attached to their partners when they feel little love for themselves. Though this is fueled by the twisted concepts mentioned above, not everyone who thinks this way becomes overly needy. But some do act out, believing that love is selfish and that their partner should give in to their every demand. Such a relationship is based on emotional instability, drama, and constant placating of the person's demands.

Strong Emotions: Though I mentioned that the sacral chakra is the primary storehouse of emotions, the heart chakra is a second-place contender for this role. Many emotions are linked to problems with relationships and issues of self-love, so people with heart chakra blockages often manifest strong and uncontrollable emotions as their heart chakra Shadow. As with previous chakras, they may lack the self-awareness to realize they have an emotional problem and, as a result, they take out their emotional pain on others.

Addiction: It's well known that addiction plagues our society. Thousands of people die every year from addiction to drugs or alcohol, and millions more are slowly killing themselves through their addictions. These substances numb the pain in the heart chakra when it is closed off, which tricks people into thinking they don't have to work to heal themselves. Unfortunately, these substances only worsen the pain and amplify any other Shadow behaviors that manifest from a closed heart chakra (such as those mentioned earlier in this section).

Now that you know how the Shadow manifests through the heart chakra, I want to reiterate this chakra's vital connection to the Shadow. As I mentioned at the beginning of this chapter, the heart is especially important because self-love and forgiveness are necessary for this process. You will struggle to fully heal yourself until you have learned to love the flaws and blind spots in your psyche. You also need to learn to forgive those who may have contributed to these problems, as they were only operating from their own Shadow.

Knowing this, you may be guided to start healing your heart chakra before any others. However, I still believe the best route is to start with the root chakra because if your lower chakras are blocked, you won't receive the energy necessary to unblock your heart chakra. Hopefully you'll agree that I've adequately outlined how the core issues of each chakra connect to one another. For example, you can't focus on pleasure (sacral chakra) until your basic needs are met (root chakra). This is why I recommend healing from the bottom up. But if you are strongly guided to start else-where (such as the heart chakra), then feel free to follow your intuition.

HEALING METHODS AND TOOLS TO UNBLOCK YOUR HEART CHAKRA

As you can tell, healing the heart chakra is one of the most important things you can do. Along the way, you will need some tools and practices to help you. Below are lists of crystals, essential oils, and foods that will help you along on your healing journey.

Crystals

The best crystals will emit the bright colors of the heart chakra (green or pink) and help you with forgiveness, self-love, and unconditional love. Below are some of the most common crystals people use to heal their heart chakra.

- **Rose Quartz:** A lovely pink quartz that aids the healing of all matters of the heart and promotes self-love and compassion.
- **Emerald:** A stunning lustrous green gem that attracts love, promotes unconditional love, and heals all negative emotions felt in the heart.
- **Green Aventurine:** A light green stone that attracts luck and heals negative emotions.
- **Rhodochrosite:** A rose-colored stone that integrates spiritual and physical energies to maintain perfect balance. It helps heal fear and trauma and encourages kindness, friendship, love, and harmony.
- **Jade:** A lustrous green gem that brings emotional balance and releases tension.
- **Malachite:** A beautiful green gem that heals and transmutes all emotional pain.
- **Amazonite:** This bluish-gray stone helps heal all past trauma and current negative emotions. It helps dissolve the blockages of your heart to allow for more kindness, trust, and love.
- **Prehnite:** A calming translucent green stone that promotes unconditional love and harmony.

Essential Oils

The best oils for the heart chakra get you in touch with your sense of self-love and encourage positive feelings.

Some of the best oils that will encourage a more loving and forgiving mindset include:

- Rose
- Jasmine
- Lavender
- Neroli
- Orange
- Sandalwood
- Ylang Ylang
- Bergamot

Diet

The best diet for healing the heart chakra includes any food that matches the green vibrancy of this chakra or promotes self-love with its nutrition. Some examples include:

- Green tea
- Green juices
- Lettuce
- Broccoli
- Kale
- Spinach
- Celery
- Zucchini

- Avocado
- Mint
- Spirulina
- Peas
- Lime
- Green apples

For an extra punch, consider blending some of these ingredients together to have a super healing ultra-heartful green smoothie.

EXERCISES FOR HEALING THE HEART CHAKRA

Healing the Shadow of the heart chakra may be far more difficult than the healing conducted in previous chapters. But it is absolutely necessary and can bring profound progress to integrating your Shadow. Below are some journal prompts, affirmations, yoga poses, and a visualization that will help you with this healing process.

Please keep in mind that healing the Shadow at this stage may result in some strong emotions and reactions. Be gentle with yourself during the process, and take time for self-care. If your feelings become too overwhelming, I recommend talking with a therapist who can help you with the process.

Journal Prompts

When journaling for the heart chakra, it's important to figure out what is hurting your relationships and sense of self-love so that you can heal those aspects of your life.

The following prompts can help you get started.

- How can I show myself unconditional love in my daily life?
- Who am I withholding forgiveness from? What do I need to let go of?
- In what ways am I too hard on myself? How can I show myself more compassion?
- What are ten things I love about myself?
- How can I show more love to the people I care about?
- What past hurts am I still holding onto?
- What is holding me back from finding love and friends?
- What do I need to do to bring more balance to my life?
- What does self-love mean to me?
- In what ways is it difficult to express intimacy? Do I have issues trusting and connecting with others?

Affirmations

Affirmations can help you let down your guard, embrace vulnerability, and dissolve the walls you've built around your heart. Negative self-talk often perpetuates our low self-worth, so the best way to heal your heart chakra is by being more loving with your thoughts and words. Below are some affirmations that will help you boost your self-love talk.

- I am worthy of love.
- I am loved.
- There is an infinite supply of love.
- I live in balance.
- I forgive myself.
- I forgive all others.
- I love myself unconditionally.
- My heart is open.
- I am healing from all past hurts.
- I deserve to be in a loving relationship.
- I create loving and supportive relationships.
- I find love everywhere I go.
- I am surrounded by wonderful and supportive people.
- I give love with ease.
- I am enough.
- I let go of all negative experiences.

- My life is in complete balance.
- I am ready to move forward with my life.
- My heart is softening.
- I am happy and free.

Yoga

When doing yoga to heal the heart chakra, you want to try poses that will open up your chest and encourage you to fully connect with your body. The following poses can help you do just that.

I must warn you, however, that many people who do these poses (or similar poses) find themselves releasing emotions very suddenly. So be gentle with yourself as you conduct your yoga sequence, and feel free to stop if you need to.

- **Bhujangasana (Cobra Pose):** Lie flat on your stomach and raise your upper body slowly, so your torso is off the ground. Try to stretch through this pose as much as possible, looking up towards the ceiling if possible. Really open your chest to receive the most healing for the heart chakra.
- **Marjaryasana / Bitilasana (Cat/Cow Poses):** Get down on all fours into a tabletop position.

Inhale, then round your back up and drop your head towards the ground. Exhale and move your head up towards the sky while curving your back inward towards the ground. Do this as many times as you feel necessary.

- **Ustrasana (Camel Pose):** Sit on your knees and lean all the way back until your neck is facing the ceiling. Grab your feet to finalize this pose.

- **Salamba Bhujangasana (Sphinx Pose):** Lie flat on your stomach and slowly raise your upper body so your chest is off the ground. Don't rise as much as you do with the cobra pose, though. Your arms should be resting at a 90 degree angle at the elbows, and your shoulders should be back so that your chest is fully open.

- **Anjaneyasana (Low Lunge Pose):** From a standing position, move into a lunge, with one leg at a 90 degree angle and the other lying flat behind your body. Once centered, lift your arms straight up to the sky with the palms facing each other.

VISUALIZATION MEDITATION

Find a comfortable spot to sit or lie down. Since healing your heart chakra can be quite an emotional endeavor, it is important to begin the session by breathing deeply for serenity and grounding. Remember to come back to your breath to process those emotions and restore your sense of calm.

Once relaxed, visualize a bright green light emitting from the center of your chest. This is your heart chakra, and it is ready to bring you love and heal your emotional pain. Feel it swirling in your chest, unblocking all the negative energy and cobwebs that keep your heart closed off. Feel the walls of your heart melting and the release of joy and love that comes when your heart is free.

This is where you may begin to feel emotional. All blockages need to be released energetically, and this often comes in the form of strong emotions for people with blocked heart chakras. You may also feel some tension or tightness in your chest. Don't push yourself to heal too quickly; do whatever you need to do for self-care. Unblocking any chakra has side effects, but the heart chakra can have some of the most painful. If you're feeling emotional, take time to breathe deeply and relax while processing your emotions.

When you feel your heart chakra unlocking and are ready to continue, visualize this green light surrounding your body. You can also visualize it as a pink light, as this is another color associated with the heart chakra. Allow this light to bask over you and hold you. You are loved. You are safe. You are lovable. Repeat these mantras if you wish, or just enjoy being held and healed by this comforting light.

Whenever you are ready, end the session by visualizing the light returning to your heart. It will always be there to heal and comfort you when you need it. Thank it for its help, and take a few more breaths. When finished with your session, slowly open your eyes.

7

THE THROAT CHAKRA (VISHUDDHA)

Color: Blue
Organs: Throat, Neck, Jaw, Mouth
Location: Throat
Element: Sound
Mantra: Ham
Planet: Mercury
Animals: White Elephant, Whale, Wolf, Bird

Now that we've healed the earthly matters governed by the lower chakras, it's time to attend to the more spiritual matters of the upper chakras. The first matter is self-expression and communication. We cannot fully connect with the Divine nor fulfill our Purpose if we struggle to communicate or express ourselves. And let's not forget, communication keeps civilization together and encourages all forms of relationships to thrive. It is challenging to navigate the world without some form of communication. For help with this, we turn to the throat chakra.

Healthy communication is something few of us master. Many are too shy to communicate effectively, while others scream and shout, desperate to be heard. But healthy communication means boldly asserting your thoughts, wants, and needs without being disrespectful to others. It requires attentive listening. Let's explore how a balanced throat chakra (also known as Vishuddha) can help with these matters.

LESSONS AND THEMES OF THE THROAT CHAKRA

The throat chakra primarily governs anything to do with speaking or expression. On the journey through the upper chakras and spirituality, it is vital to have the courage and ability to express yourself. The lower chakras help you define who you are; the throat chakra helps you communicate your identity to the world.

Let's take a look at how the throat chakra helps with this.

Communication: As mentioned, the main theme of the throat chakra is communication. Communication is the primary way our species interacts with one another. Humans have developed languages and multiple forms of communication that keep our relationships rich and civilizations complex. Without a healthy throat chakra, we may stumble on our words, not know what to say, or lack the confidence to speak at all.

Speaking Your Truth: The throat chakra is the chakra of honesty. It helps you to speak your truth and be honest in every way. Honesty takes courage and inner power. It's not always easy to tell the truth or stand for what you believe in. But a healthy chakra can help you maintain this power and courage.

Self-Expression: Communication is also essential for self-expression. Without communication, no one would know much about us; our needs, wants, desires, personality, etc. Whether verbally or nonverbally, we use communication to tell the world who we are, what we want and need, and what makes us unique. The throat chakra is crucial to clearly expressing oneself, and is the only way the world knows who we are.

Listening: We can't have good communication without good listening. People today often don't know how to listen in conversations. Instead of listening to what is being said, they simply wait for opportunities to contribute to the conversation. Many of us struggle in conversation when we are not the ones talking, but a healthy throat chakra can help you become a better listener and overall conversationalist.

Inner Voice: The throat chakra governs not only our physical voice but our inner voice as well. This inner voice often acts as our conscience or cheerleader but can also be the source of negative self-talk when encumbered by the Shadow.

COMMON REASONS THE THROAT CHAKRA BECOMES BLOCKED

The right to speak and express oneself is a right that everyone should have, but few are able to experience. Even in the "free world," many people feel powerless, and are dissuaded from speaking their truth. Let's take a look at the most common ways the throat chakra becomes blocked and why you may not feel comfortable speaking out or being assertive.

Shame or Guilt: People with something to hide don't want witnesses to speak out against them, so will threaten, shame, or guilt people from speaking. We were all witness to the power such threatening actions had when the #MeToo movement began. For decades, women were too intimidated to speak out against sexual harassment in the workplace. They were often threatened with being fired or having their careers ruined if they did not remain silent. Many women were even shamed for being in such circumstances in the first place, even when they didn't have the power to protect themselves. Not being allowed to speak about these situations can make a woman feel insignificant in a world run by men, so her energy contracts inside and blocks her throat chakra.

Verbal Abuse: Verbal abuse can be just as detrimental as physical abuse. It is used to emotionally break down the victim and make them feel powerless and insignificant. Victims of verbal abuse often feel overpowered by their abusers, which causes them to unconsciously shut down their own voices.

Being Forced to Keep Secrets: When we are forced to keep secrets or hide information, we are blocked from expressing our full inner truth. The secret can be as mundane as not telling a guy that your friend has a crush on him or as serious as being threatened into remaining silent about the sexual abuse you experienced as a child. When forced to keep secrets, we hold information back, which causes an energetic blockage.

Receiving Mixed Messages: When people give us mixed messages, it makes communication confusing. For example, if someone tells us they like us but then engages in activities that we feel are sabotaging us, we're bound to be confused about their true intentions. Mixed messages that cause significant emotional damage may erode our trust in other people, as it will be harder to trust anyone's words when we've been on the receiving end of many lies.

Not Allowed to Speak During Childhood: If a person wasn't allowed to speak out in childhood, they will be afraid to speak out in adulthood. Controlling and authoritarian parents who don't listen to or allow their children to speak their minds unconsciously tell their children that their needs and their self-expression do not matter. A person with this inner messaging will struggle to communicate efficiently in adulthood because they tend to believe their needs aren't important.

Not Being Heard: If you were ever in a situation in which you weren't heard or were deliberately ignored, then you'll be dissuaded from participating in future conversations. These situations occur primarily in abusive relationships or when we're surrounded by people who have little to no respect for us. When people consistently show they don't care about what you have to say, it can make you feel like your words aren't important enough to share with anyone else, causing a blockage.

SIGNS OF AN IMBALANCED THROAT CHAKRA

When we can't communicate properly, we struggle to meet our own needs and have fulfilling connections with others. These struggles can lead to mental health concerns, physical ailments, and other life challenges. Below are lists of the common issues people with imbalanced throat chakras often live with.

Common emotional and mental health concerns that arise from a blocked throat chakra include:

- Social anxiety
- Compulsive lying
- Loneliness from being unheard
- Low self-esteem
- Anger management concerns
- Social phobias or phobias concerning social settings
- Negative self-talk that can lead to depression, anxiety, and other mental health concerns

Common physical ailments that develop from a blocked throat chakra include:

- Chronic sore throat
- Gum disease
- Mouth ulcers
- Laryngitis
- Thyroid issues
- Raspy throat
- Sinus problems
- Respiratory problems

Life challenges that manifest from a blocked throat chakra include:

- Trouble telling the truth or speaking one's inner truth
- Issues with public speaking
- Passive aggressive behavior and communication
- Unable to communicate effectively in relationships
- Compulsive or pathological lying
- Having a quiet voice
- Constant complaining or negative talk
- Difficulty expressing ideas or thoughts
- Yelling and shouting to be heard

THE THROAT CHAKRA AND THE SHADOW

When the Shadow manifests in the throat chakra, we develop an unhealthy communication style. We interact with people in ways that eventually make it clear to them that we either can't be trusted or will not respect them. This behavior can manifest in a myriad of ways:

Lying: When people are afraid of the truth, they create lies to deceive others. These lies prevent others from discovering the truth and from seeing the person's weaknesses, flaws, or misbehaviors. Lies are told by those who know they are doing wrong and/or feels insecure with who they are. Even more innocent or understandable lies (such as lying about your sexuality if you live in an area where it is shamed) are a manifestation of the Shadow because they come from your shame and insecurity (even if it is understandable).

Persecuting Others Who Do Speak Out: Liars often persecute those who choose to tell the truth. Whether it be a child who tells the teacher who stole a classmate's pencil or a whistleblower exposing the unethical actions of a tech company, those who dare to speak out are often persecuted and harassed by those who wish for the information to remain a secret. Keeping the secret helps the person feel safe and secure, even if it is wrong and unethical. They feel threatened when others find out the truth about them and their misdeeds.

Passive Aggressive Communication: When the Shadow manifests in the throat chakra, we feel insecure directly admitting the truth. We are likely to develop more passive-aggressive language and tactics to make the truth known without directly stating it. This kind of communication can manifest as gossip, sarcasm, mumbling under one's breath, or subtle forms of sabotage.

Not Listening: When we have a blocked throat chakra, we become obsessed with how people perceive us. Therefore, one way or another, we curate our language and communication skills to craft the perception we want. All this effort makes it difficult to listen to others. We are so focused on how we are perceived in a conversation that we don't listen to what others are saying. Some people even develop a habit of only listening for things they can use to control the conversation.

Yelling and Screaming: When people feel unheard or unseen, they will sometimes become louder and louder until everyone finally listens. They feel they need to be louder and more demanding because, internally, they feel small and insignificant. This may stem from feeling unheard or being exposed to shouting and yelling as a child. But this behavior only perpetuates the cycle. This individual is only heard because they silence others with their shouting, not because they are respected or loved.

Verbal Abuse: When we are insecure, we find methods to control others so we can feel powerful. Those with issues and a Shadow in the throat chakra may develop communication to control others. This usually manifests as verbal abuse, which can take the form of blaming, shaming, criticizing, gaslighting, or demeaning.

Anger Issues: When you feel unheard or ignored, what emotion do you typically feel? You probably feel anger, or at least irritation. People who have Shadow issues in the throat chakra feel consistently unheard (or at least disrespected) for one reason or another. If they can't find a productive way to express themselves and be heard to their satisfaction, they may develop chronic anger issues, and could take these issues out on others in the form of verbal abuse, yelling, or shouting.

Negative Self-Talk: It is important to mention that Shadow issues connected to the throat chakra can also affect how we talk to ourselves. Dealing with adverse experiences like verbal abuse or harsh criticism can easily influence our inner monologue. If the Shadow does not manifest in your communication style with others, then it may show up in how you think and speak about yourself. This inner monologue often contains the words of your former abusers or critics that you haven't healed from.

HEALING METHODS AND TOOLS TO UNBLOCK YOUR THROAT CHAKRA

Without a healthy throat chakra, you won't be able to communicate your wants and needs adequately in life. You may resort to passive-aggressive behavior, extremely aggressive communication, or just be flat-out passive. This throat chakra needs balancing in order to establish positive communication. Below are some healing methods that can help.

Crystals

When looking for crystals that heal the throat chakra, seek out those that help with communication, give you the courage to speak your truth, and improve your negative self-talk. A few options are listed below.

- **Amazonite:** A teal-colored crystal that heals trauma, worry, and fear, so you can courageously speak your truth.
- **Lapis Lazuli:** A stunning blue stone that helps heal repressed emotions and encourages self-awareness. It also helps you to discover your

needs and wants and communicate them effectively.

- **Turquoise:** A turquoise gem that facilitates and unblocks all forms of communication.
- **Aquamarine:** A lovely aquamarine gem that connects the heart to the throat chakra, allowing your deepest truths to be felt and expressed.
- **Sodalite:** Another gorgeous dark blue stone that helps you express your thoughts clearly and unblocks any energy preventing your creativity. It particularly helps artists and performers gain confidence and improve their communication skills.
- **Blue Kyanite:** A blue gemstone that cuts through fears and promotes courage to help one speak their truth. It also aids with public speaking and performing.
- **Blue Lace Agate:** A sky blue stone that neutralizes negative emotions that block the throat chakra (such as anger) and encourages the expression of thoughts and feelings.

Essential Oils

The best essential oils are those that help stimulate and air out the sinuses and respiratory system. Problems with these areas of the body often make it difficult to speak, as they prevent your body from getting enough oxygen to communicate effectively. Below are a few essential oils that can help with this.

- Frankincense
- Rosemary
- Eucalyptus
- Tea tree
- Peppermint
- Spearmint
- Basil

Diet

When changing your diet for the throat chakra, you want foods that do two things: 1) exhibit the same blue hue as the chakra itself and 2) soothe and heal the throat. There are numerous healthy foods that do this, including:

- Blueberries
- Blackberries
- Blue corn

- Coconut water
- Raw honey
- Herbal teas
- Lemons
- Apples
- Pears

Vocal Exercises

Since the throat chakra is all about using your voice, one of the best ways to unblock it is by being vocal. There are many ways you can do this, including singing, chanting, and toning.

You can also use seed mantras, which are mantras that have specific spiritual powers. Each chakra has an associated mantra that helps unblock it, and seed mantras are particularly powerful for healing the throat chakra. The seed mantra for the throat chakra is *Ham*. Affirmations are also quite powerful for healing the throat chakra, as I say below.

EXERCISES FOR HEALING THE THROAT CHAKRA

In addition to the tools mentioned, I've also provided some shadow work exercises that will help you unblock your throat chakra and integrate this part of your Shadow.

Journal Prompts

When journaling for the throat chakra, you want to analyze how your communication style and habits present you as a person. Do you come off as a liar or drama queen? Do people think you're too shy or timid? Or do people have a healthy respect for you because you tactfully assert your needs and boundaries? Keep these questions in mind as you answer the following journal prompts:

- How do I communicate in conversations? How much do I spend listening compared to speaking? Is this ratio balanced?
- How do I communicate with other people? Do I speak truthfully, or do I lie to please others?
- What does authenticity mean to me?
- What can I do to feel more confident when speaking in social situations?
- When I encounter lies and gossip, how can I respond in a calm and effective way?
- What "white lies" do I often tell, and why do I tell them?

- Are there situations when I feel like I'm faking my persona or forcing myself to be someone else? How do I feel when I do this?
- Do I keep my word? What can I do to keep more of my promises?
- How do I feel when I meet someone who has no problem being their authentic self? Do I admire them, or do I feel threatened?
- How can I become a better listener?

Affirmations

Affirmations are a particularly powerful healing option for the throat chakra, considering they utilize the voice and throat. When using affirmations for the throat chakra, you want to empower yourself to improve your communication style and affirm your ability to speak the truth. Below are a few affirmations that will help you with these concerns.

- I hear and speak the truth.
- I am truthful and honest in all my communication.
- I express myself with clear intent.
- I let my voice be heard.
- I express my creativity with ease.
- I do no harm with my words.
- I speak with authenticity and courage.

- I always speak my inner truth.
- I always act on my inner truth.
- I can speak in public with calm and ease.
- I speak confidently in front of others.
- I speak my truth lovingly.
- I uplift others with my words.
- I speak and listen with equal awareness.
- I listen with compassion and understanding.
- I balance my speech and actions with deep listening.
- I always make my intent clear.
- I am not afraid to ask for what I want and need.
- I effectively communicate my boundaries.
- My voice is necessary.

Yoga Poses

To clear the throat chakra using yoga, look for poses that will stretch the throat, neck, and shoulder areas. Below are a few that will help.

Bhujangasana (Cobra Pose): Lie flat on your stomach and raise your upper body slowly, so your torso is off the ground. Try to stretch through this pose as much as possible as you look towards the ceiling.

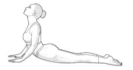

Ustrasana (Camel Pose): Sit on your knees and lean all the way back until your neck is facing the ceiling. Grab your feet to finalize this pose.

Matsyasana (Fish Pose): Lie on your back with your legs straight. Bend your elbows back so your forearms are on the floor, then lift your chest toward the ceiling. Rest on the crown of your head while keeping your chest lifted.

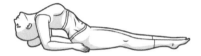

Simhasana (Lion's Breath): Get on your knees, spread them apart and lean forward on all fours. Lift your chest and head up, then open your mouth and stick out your tongue like a dog.

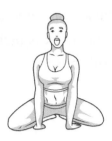

Salama Sarvangasana (Shoulderstand): This is a more advanced pose for people with great torso strength or who have been yogis for a long time. From a lying position, slowly lift up your legs until they are pointing toward the ceiling. Now lift your torso off the ground. The goal is for your whole body to be held up by your neck and shoulders.

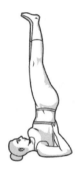

VISUALIZATION MEDITATION

Find a comfortable spot to sit or lie down. Begin with some deep breathing to ground and calm yourself. Pay particular attention to your breath. Notice how it flows in and out, either through your nose or mouth. Allow all tension to be released through every exhale. Continue this until you feel deeply relaxed.

Now, bring your attention to a blue light glowing in your throat. Notice the brilliant blue light it emits and how it feels. Do you feel tension in your throat, as though your words and thoughts are struggling to get out? Or does the energy feel free? Take note of any sensations you experience.

Allow this blue light to swirl and clear out any blockages. Once your throat feels unblocked, allow the blue light to cover your entire neck or even your full head or body if you wish. This light is giving you the power to speak your truth. There is no reason to hide or act small. You are safe and have the power to speak your mind. You deserve to speak up and be heard.

While absorbing the healing of the blue light, feel free to say any affirmations or mantras that come to mind. You can also chant, hum, or sing. Any form of vocal expression is welcome here. If you have the sudden urge to say something or vocalize, that means your soul is crying out to be heard. What does it want to say? Take note of the words and affirmations your soul longs to speak.

When you are finished, allow the energy to condense again to your throat. Know that it will always be available to help you with all matters of communication. Thank your throat chakra for being the communication gateway of your soul and for giving you the power to speak. Take a few more breaths and slowly open your eyes.

8

THE THIRD EYE CHAKRA (AJNA)

Color: Indigo
Organs: Eyes, Pineal Gland
Location: Brow
Element: Light
Mantra: Om
Planet: Saturn
Animals: Owl, Cat

Whereas the last chakra dealt with matters relating to sound, we now move to the chakra that governs all matters of sight. Sight is one of the most important senses we have. Having the gift of physical sight makes the world much easier to navigate. But sight isn't just a physical sense. Spiritual sight (such as in the forms of clairvoyance and dreams) allows us to peek into the spiritual realm and interact with meta-physical beings. And there is also mental sight (which can manifest as wisdom, intuition, or inner vision), which helps us see through illusions and visualize a path for our future. The third eye chakra governs the energy of all these forms.

The third eye chakra (also known as Ajna) is the chakra that many spiritual seekers spend the most time healing and opening. It governs so many matters essential for enlightenment that it's no wonder people become preoccupied with it. It helps us develop our intuition and wisdom, guides us on our spiritual path, and helps us discover and develop our spiritual gifts. It also helps us see ourselves with full self-awareness and increases our trust in ourselves and our instincts. It's the first chakra so far with a dominant influence in spiritual matters. Let's now review all the ways this important chakra influences our life and spiritual path.

LESSONS AND THEMES OF THE THIRD EYE CHAKRA

Once again, the third eye chakra covers almost everything to do with the concept of sight. Sight is not just physical vision, though; it also includes spiritual and mental sight.

Below are the overarching themes and matters influenced by the third eye chakra.

Intuition: Intuition is the unconscious recognition of patterns. It is a combination of mental insight and communication with Spirit. Intuition is one of the most desired spiritual gifts, as it helps us stay on our path and see opportunities that the rational brain would overlook. However, intuition is passive and can't be forced. The only ways to improve intuition are to be more open and relaxed and to keep your spiritual eye open to opportunities and signs.

Dreams: Dreams are often a window into the soul. They come with imagery and messages that indicate subconscious fears, desires, and needs. Dreams are also used as a form of communication with Spirit; many people receive life-changing spiritual messages through their dreams. When the third eye is open, it can receive these messages easier. When it's closed, you may forget your dreams entirely.

Visualization and Imagination: Your imagination and ability to visualize are essential on the path to attaining your life purpose and designing your ideal life. Without these gifts, you cannot see the road ahead nor have a clue where your life is going. These gifts are also important if you wish to have a creative hobby or career. The third eye must be wide open for these gifts to be optimized.

Vision: The term "vision" refers to multiple concepts. Of course, the third eye can affect matters regarding physical vision and tangible issues with the eyes. But someone with vision has a grand dream for their future and plans to reach their goals. Most of us need physical vision to navigate the world, and everyone needs a grand vision of their life to feel fulfilled and feel as if they have a purpose.

Insight: Having the gift of insight helps us cut through the illusions and deceptions of modern society and see situations as they truly are. Without this awareness, we are more susceptible to deception and manipulation. Insight keeps us on the right path and prevents us from being with the wrong people or becoming involved in bad situations.

Self-Awareness: The greatest form of sight that anyone can develop is self-awareness. Too many people, whether consciously or unconsciously, block their awareness. As a result, they have an inaccurate image of themselves, which often takes the forms of narcissism or self-degradation. Without awareness, we cannot work to minimize our faults or have an accurate understanding of our strengths. Self-awareness is also critical to doing any shadow work, as I will explain later in the chapter.

Spiritual Gifts: In addition to intuition, the third eye chakra helps us enhance and develop other spiritual gifts. This can include clairvoyance, precognition, and imagination. Furthermore, the third eye is often thought of as the seat of wisdom, which in my opinion is the best spiritual gift of all.

COMMON REASONS THE THIRD EYE CHAKRA BECOMES BLOCKED

Since humans are typically more focused on earthly matters, it is very common for the upper chakras to be deficient or blocked. People usually focus on the here and now so much that they rarely develop their spiritual gifts and overall vision for their lives. Though staying in the present is usually a good thing, not having any insight or plan for the future can hinder your spiritual and physical progress on this planet.

It doesn't help that this is a difficult planet to navigate, where deceit, illusion, heartbreak, and betrayal are hard to avoid. Interacting with anyone who questions your talent, abilities, or inherent self-worth can make you question yourself and hide the gifts that make you unique.

Below are some common ways this can happen.

Repressed Memories/Trauma: We cannot fully know who we are if we don't remember everything we have been through. When we block memories, no matter how traumatic, we block a part of ourselves. We cannot have complete awareness or experience integration without bringing these memories to light. When we repress memories, even subconsciously, we turn a blind eye to certain aspects of our lives and ourselves. Working in therapy to remember and heal these memories can restore our insight and self-awareness.

Shame: When we are shamed for who we are, we lose trust in our instincts and path. Even if you have strongly developed spiritual and psychic gifts, you may not trust yourself to use them. Furthermore, you will lack the trust and self-worth needed to create a grander vision of your life and protect yourself from illusions and deceit.

Frightening and Traumatizing Environments: There are some things that, once seen, cannot be unseen. A single traumatic visual (such as images from war or a gruesome crime) can traumatize a person for life. People who see something frightening or have been exposed to traumatic and frightening environments (such as an abusive home or a war zone) often carry that trauma throughout their lives. These situations subconsciously encourage a person to shut down their sight to prevent similar experiences in the future. Though a person rarely loses their physical sight, their mental sight (such as their vision for their future) and spiritual sight (such as clairvoyance or other spiritual gifts) are often compromised.

Lack of Spiritual Life: It's easy to become so hyper-focused on the day-to-day grind that we fail to incorporate spiritual elements into our routines. But having a spiritual life allows us to tend to our souls, which are often neglected as we focus on more earthly matters. A spiritual life also allows us to connect to something greater than ourselves, whether it be Spirit or humanity as a whole.

This doesn't mean you need to follow New Age philosophies to have an open third eye. Spiritual life includes anything that fills your soul. It can be a life filled with creativity or a life devoted to God and prayer. A spiritual life can also include service, volunteer work, or dedicating your life to a specific cause.

Fear: Having any type of fear, whether from trauma, a phobia, or something else, can shut down our mental or spiritual vision. When we fear something, we don't want to look at it. In the context of mental and spiritual sight, if we are afraid of our spiritual gifts or their repercussions, we may close them off from ourselves.

For example, a person afraid of ridicule she may get for doing tarot readings may shut down her intuition and communication with Spirit through her third eye.

Adverse Spiritual/Religious Experiences: Many people are walking away from religion and spirituality because of negative experiences, which is perfectly understandable. Certain spiritual and religious groups are trying to drag the world backward with their traditional and discriminatory beliefs. This leads to frightening situations affecting millions of people worldwide. As a result, people may cut off all connections to spirituality because they see it as a bad thing. While it's understandable that people walk away, the truth is that certain traditions or faiths are not inherently corrupt, but have simply been corrupted by specific individuals. The wickedness of the few shouldn't necessitate a complete blocking off of spirituality.

SIGNS OF AN IMBALANCED THIRD EYE CHAKRA

Because the third eye chakra controls much regarding physical and spiritual sight, numerous problems can occur if this chakra is blocked or imbalanced. For example, a blocked third eye can cause self-awareness and self-image issues, which can significantly alter one's mental health. A blockage in the third eye can also affect health concerns such as issues regarding physical eyesight. And, of course, life is far more challenging if we do not have good intuition and insight to guide us. Below are some of the common mental health concerns, physical ailments, and life challenges that arise when this chakra is out of alignment.

Emotional and mental health concerns of the third eye chakra include:

- Poor memory
- Difficulty concentrating
- Hallucinations
- Depression
- Anxiety
- Severe psychological disorders (e.g., schizophrenia)
- Living in denial
- Losing touch with reality
- Narcissism

Physical ailments tied to the third eye chakra include:

- Poor vision or other issues regarding the eyes
- Headaches
- Issues with the pineal gland
- Brain concerns and disorders

Life challenges that manifest from a blocked third eye chakra include:

- Lack of imagination
- Disconnect from spiritual gifts
- Poor dream recall
- Difficulty envisioning the future
- Nightmares
- Difficulty processing information
- Struggling to plan for the future
- Underactive imagination
- Lack of a clear path in life
- No goals or motivators
- Indulging in escapism
- Rejection of all spirituality
- Indecisiveness
- Lack of self-awareness
- Feeling stuck without solutions to life challenges

THE THIRD EYE CHAKRA AND THE SHADOW

Just as with the heart chakra, the third eye chakra is particularly important when it comes to the concept of the Shadow. In order to integrate the Shadow, we must have self-awareness and clear insight. Without these, we fail to recognize our flaws, limiting beliefs, and shortcomings. This hinders our growth and healing and keeps us blind to who we truly are. But integration is all about knowing and loving our full self, so we need to heal the third eye chakra in order to succeed with Shadow integration.

As you might imagine, the ways in which the Shadow manifests through the third eye all relate to vision and insight. People who have these Shadow issues fail to see themselves and their situations accurately. Below are some common ways this can manifest.

Denial: With a blocked third eye, we cannot see who we really are. We are blind to our true selves and choose to remain blind even when everyone else can see us clearly.

People in denial do not want to admit their flaws, so they behave as though they don't have them. Psychology explains that this a defense mechanism to protect ourselves from experiencing insecurities or uncomfortable emotions. People in denial refuse to develop a clear self-image because it is too painful for them.

Though we all experience some level of denial at some point in our lives, severe and chronic denial can make it seem as though a person is not in touch with reality. Others can see the flaws or a situation clearly, but the person in denial cannot. The result is that denial often causes far more problems than it prevents.

It's also important to note that projection is often connected to denial. A person in denial about their flaws will project them onto other people. For example, someone in denial about their anger may insist that other people around them have an anger problem. Projection is another defense mechanism, and it is used to shift the blame to someone else. It requires denying reality and being blind to your true self.

Dreams: If the Shadow cannot reach you through the pain it causes and messages it sends you during waking hours, then it will try to reach you while you are asleep. While sleeping, you cannot actively deny reality or fight against the truth, so it's easier for your mind and for Spirit to communicate with you during this time. For this reason, while healing your Shadow (whether focusing on the third eye or other chakras), I encourage you to do dreamwork and dream journaling. These activities can help you explore messages delivered to you while you are asleep.

Lack of Self-Awareness: It's one thing to deny that a situation happened; it is another to have no understanding of who you are and how people perceive you. We all have specific visions in our heads of who we think we are. When reality corrects this vision, some of us choose to accept it while others choose to deny it. Self-awareness is essential for spiritual maturity and emotional well-being. If you can't face who you are, you will never love and accept your true self.

A lack of self-awareness is often tied to deep insecurity. Insecurity is painful, and forces us to confront the fact that we aren't perfect. This isn't easy for anyone, and some choose to turn a blind eye to their true selves. Unfortunately, lack of self-awareness can be dangerous and even contributes to toxic personality traits and disorders such as Narcissistic Personality Disorder.

Attachment to an Illusion or Image: We all know that person who has a specific vision for what every human should do and does not waiver from it. For example, they may think that humans should stick to clearly defined gender roles or that everyone should have a specific career path. The image or vision they have of themselves and everyone else is all they have to relieve them from their insecurities. But it's not enough that they maintain this narrow vision in their own lives; they also project it onto others. More often than not, this state of mind is accompanied by a lack of self-awareness. These people don't realize that not only are other people more dimensional than their vision allows, but that they themselves don't perfectly fit into the delusion they've created for themselves. It is often the most flawed people who force others to be their version of perfect.

Shaming and Discrimination of Religion and Spiritual Paths: People with Shadow issues in the third eye are not only completely disconnected from their spiritual life but are uncomfortable with others who have one. They are highly focused on physical matters so they think everyone else should be too. This is often triggered by insecurities regarding spirituality or past adverse experiences with religion.

This trait does not exist only in atheists and agnostics. When religious people discriminate against other religions, they are showing the Shadow sides of their spiritual lives. There is a deep insecurity that governs the belief that only one religious path is the true path. Hatred or vitriol towards another religion is the Shadow trying to show itself through the third eye chakra.

HEALING METHODS AND TOOLS TO UNBLOCK YOUR THIRD EYE CHAKRA

Developing our spiritual gifts and restoring our physical and spiritual vision is critical for success in the physical and spiritual realms. Without a healthy third eye chakra, we cannot see where we are headed or navigate situations with wisdom and insight, which makes this a very important chakra to heal. Below are lists of crystals, essential oils, and foods that can help with healing.

Crystals

The best crystals for the third eye chakra are stones that exhibit the beautiful indigo shades of the chakra and help with your spiritual gifts, intuition, and insight. Below are some of the most common crystals used for healing the third eye.

- **Lapis Lazuli:** A stunning dark blue and gold stone that helps you connect with your intuition, insight, and inner wisdom.
- **Sodalite:** A striking blue and white stone that calms the mind and supports self-acceptance and awareness.
- **Violet Tourmaline:** A lovely violet stone that supports spiritual growth and problem-solving.
- **Fluorite:** A gorgeous gemstone that comes in a wide variety of blues, greens, and purples. This crystal helps promote spiritual awakening, intuition, and other psychic gifts.
- **Celestite:** A lovely sky-blue stone that helps with wisdom, mindfulness, and higher consciousness. It also helps calm the mind of

negative emotions and stress so you can better connect with your intuition.

- **Amethyst:** A beautiful purple gemstone that helps you connect with the Divine. It also brings you into a focused and relaxed state and heightens your awareness. Amethyst is also known for connecting with the unconscious mind, helping you with your dreamwork and intuition.
- **Labradorite:** A dazzling gem that exhibits all the colors of Aurora Borealis. It helps to awaken intuition and develop your psychic gifts.

Essential Oils

When choosing essential oils for the third eye chakra, you should choose those that help calm your emotions, open your spiritual gifts, and connect you with your intuition. Some oils that can help include:

- Lavender
- Clary Sage
- Rose
- Chamomile
- Frankincense
- Patchouli
- Sandalwood

Diet

When healing the third eye, you should incorporate foods that have the same purple or indigo hue as the chakra. Some examples are:

- Grapes
- Blueberries
- Lavender flavored tea
- Chocolate
- Eggplant
- Purple kale
- Purple carrots
- Plums

In addition to adding the above foods, it's important to cut out junk food if you want to heal this chakra. Sugar, additives, preservatives, etc., calcify the third eye and pineal gland, which makes it much harder for them to operate normally. So, although improving your diet is always a good idea, no matter which chakra you are working on, it is even more crucial for healing the third eye chakra.

Dream Journal

Your third eye may also benefit from writing in a dream journal. Dream journaling is often used by people who want to remember their dreams or to promote more dreaming in general.

To do this, pick your favorite journal or notebook and keep it by your bedside. In the morning when you wake up from a dream, immediately record every detail you can remember. When you are more awake, you can analyze the details to see if there are any meanings or messages in them. Doing this consistently will unveil any patterns or messages your subconscious is trying to show you. You may experience more vivid and memorable dreams as well.

EXERCISES FOR HEALING THE THIRD EYE CHAKRA

In addition to the tools mentioned, I've provided some shadow work exercises and a few other tips that will help you unblock your third eye chakra, heal your spiritual insight, and integrate this part of your Shadow.

Journal Prompts

When journaling for the third eye chakra, explore themes or past situations that keep you from seeing something clearly or prevent you from exploring your spiritual gifts.

Some example journal prompts are:

- What are my spiritual gifts? Am I using them to their fullest potential?
- In what areas of life am I open-minded? In what areas am I more stubborn or close-minded?
- What was my relationship with my imagination like when I was a kid? Was I encouraged to be imaginative or discouraged?
- What can I do each day to strengthen my intuition?
- Do I generally have the ability to see past the illusion in situations? If not, what can I do to become more insightful?
- Have there been any recurrent themes in my dreams lately? Is my soul trying to speak to me through my dreams? What is it trying to say?
- What does my vision for my future look like? What are some baby steps I can take now to make that vision a reality?
- How do I perceive myself? Does this line up with how people describe me?
- In what ways do I see things that others don't?
- Take a few minutes to visualize your perfect life. What does it look like? Describe in as much detail as possible.

Affirmations

To use affirmations for healing your third eye, find statements that connect you with your wisdom, intuition, and other spiritual gifts. It's also important to develop greater insight and vision about your surroundings. Below are some example affirmations that can help you with this.

- I see all things in clarity.
- I trust in myself.
- I am a wise being.
- I see the path ahead.
- I am fully developing my psychic gifts.
- I always trust my intuition.
- I am open to new experiences.
- I trust my instincts and my decisions.
- I am open to the wisdom within.
- I can manifest my vision.
- It is safe for me to see the truth.
- My imagination is vivid and powerful.
- I see beyond what is apparent to what is really there.
- I am connected to the wisdom of the Universe.
- I visualize myself achieving my goals.
- I am able to see and act in alignment with my divine purpose.

- I embrace my wisdom as a bridge to my higher self.
- My imagination shows me that anything is possible.
- I trust my intuition to guide me to the right path.
- My dreams give me insight into my soul's desires and path.

Yoga Poses

Yoga poses that help the third eye chakra involve resting the head and utilizing the strength of the upper body. To unblock this chakra, it's important to get energy moving from the chest up, so you should include poses that strengthen the neck and head. Below are a few that can help.

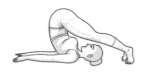

Plow Pose (Halasana): Lie down and press your arms to the floor, then lift up your legs and torso. Move your legs backward over your head and down towards the floor as if you were about to do a backward somersault.

Balasana (Child's Pose): Sit on your heels and lean forward, resting your head on the ground. Rest your arms beside your legs, palms out. For a greater stretch in the hips, move your legs further apart. You can also extend your arms out in front of you.

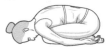

Adho Mukha Svanasana (Downward Facing Dog): From a standing position, bend forward and place your hands on the floor. Walk your legs back so your body makes a downward V-shape. Relax your head between your arms or rest it all the way on the ground if you have the flexibility.

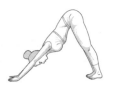

Uttanasana (Standing Forward Bend): From a standing position, lean forward and bend all the way down. Put your fingertips on the floor for support. Release your head and neck, allowing them to relax.

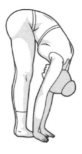

Catur Svanasana (Dolphin Pose): This pose is similar to downward facing dog, but instead of putting your hands on the floor, rest your upper body on your forearms.

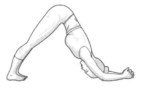

Janu Sirsasana (Head-To-Knee Pose): From a sitting position, straighten one leg and fold in the other. Grab the foot that is stretched out and bend your torso and head towards it. If you can, try to touch your head to your knee.

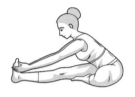

VISUALIZATION MEDITATION

Find a comfortable spot to sit or lie down. Take some slow, deep breaths to relax your body and mind. Allow the stressors and tension of the day to float away and bring yourself into a relaxed state.

When you are completely relaxed, visualize a bright indigo light shining on your forehead. This is your third eye chakra, and it wants to help you visualize and attain your dreams. Notice how the energy swirls around. Visualize this light becoming brighter as it clears out any blockages that are slowing it down. Take note of any feelings or sensations in your brow during this process.

Once your third eye is clear, take some time to visualize your dream life. What achievements have you accomplished? Who is part of your support network? How does this image make you feel? Fully immerse yourself in this dream landscape. Allow yourself to believe it is possible and that it is coming, because it is.

After you have spent some time visualizing your dream life and how you will attain it, feel free to speak any affirmations that will help you develop the gifts and talents you need to pursue this path. Notice how much more confident and connected you feel the more you unblock your third eye.

When you are ready, allow the energy to condense back to your brow. Know that it will always be available to help you connect with your soul and remember your gifts. Thank your third eye chakra for giving you insight and vision. When you are finished, take a few more breaths and slowly open your eyes.

9

THE CROWN CHAKRA
(SAHASRARA)

Color: Violet or White
Organs: Head, Brain
Location: Above the Head
Element: Thought
Mantra: Ah
Planet: Jupiter
Animals: Eagle, Bird, Butterfly

It has been a long journey, but we have finally arrived at the final chakra: the crown chakra, also known as Sahasrara. This chakra is located just above the head, acting as our gateway to the heavens. It is in charge of most spiritual matters, including consciousness, spiritual communication, and connecting to our higher self.

Since it is considered the most spiritual chakra, many people believe that focusing more on spiritual matters than earthly matters is the best way to open this chakra. However, I believe that the core lesson of this chakra is merging your consciousness with the earthly plane to create a balance. Duality is a big challenge for most humans. Some fight it by only seeking worldly pleasures, while others seek spiritual escapism. Neither path is healthy. The soul's purpose and true desire is to merge both sides of this duality so that we have a balance of earthly responsibilities and spiritual bliss.

This is why, while opening up the crown chakra can help you develop a healthy spiritual life, it's important not to go overboard and neglect your earthly responsibilities. Let's explore how the crown chakra helps us to maintain this balance and creates a spiritual life that nourishes the soul.

LESSONS AND THEMES OF THE CROWN CHAKRA

As we've learned, the crown chakra has to do with spiritual matters. But it also governs matters related to thought, intellect, and the mind.

Below are the common themes and responsibilities of the crown chakra.

Connection with Spirit: The crown chakra is our main connection to a higher power. Whether you call that higher power God, Spirit, Allah, or something else, the crown chakra helps you communicate with it. Messages from Spirit come in many forms, including clairvoyance, clairaudience, and intuitive feelings. But no matter what form of communication you use to connect with a higher power, your crown chakra helps with that connection.

Consciousness: Consciousness is your awareness that you are an infinite soul. It creates our thoughts, experiences, emotions, and connects us with the Universe. When you expand your consciousness, you become more aware of the mysteries of the Universe. The crown chakra helps you to connect with this consciousness and expand it for spiritual enlightenment.

Thought and Intellect: Since the crown chakra is closest to the brain, it also governs most issues of the mind. Intelligence, thought, and focus are all highly influenced by the energy of this chakra. It is also in charge of claircognizance, the spiritual gift of "clear knowing." When you possess this gift, you simply know certain things, even if you have no evidence to back up your knowledge. Your crown chakra is the source of your thoughts, ideas, and messages you get from claircognizance.

Belief Systems: The crown chakra is also where you store your overarching belief systems. This could relate to spirituality and religion, but non-theistic belief systems are also stored here. A healthy crown chakra usually results in belief systems that are receptive and open-minded. As we will explore later, imbalances and the Shadow contribute to harmful belief systems, but the crown chakra encourages us to examine our belief systems to determine whether or not they are limiting or harmful in any way.

Spiritual Identity: Since the crown chakra is in charge of all spiritual matters, it helps us attune to our spiritual identity. As we live on this Earth, we take on an earthly persona to navigate the world. But our true identity is our soul. Many people live lives that block their connection to their souls, but opening up the crown chakra reestablishes this connection and reminds us who we are: a divine being of light and love.

COMMON REASONS THE CROWN CHAKRA BECOMES BLOCKED

As I touched on in the last chapter, since the world is primarily focused on earthly matters, the crown chakra is often blocked for many people. Few strive to heal this chakra because society can sometimes dismiss spirituality as having little importance. But a connection to spirituality adds peace and satisfaction to an existence that may feel like it has no meaning. Below are a few of the most common situations that cause blockages in the crown chakra.

Attached to Earthly Concerns: Though being rooted in earthly matters is essential to having a solid foundation in life, this does not mean that we should ignore spiritual matters. Connecting with Spirit (as well as the global human consciousness) brings life, peace, and satisfaction to your soul. When you focus only on making money and acquiring material things, you ignore your soul, which can cause depression and a feeling of emptiness from a lack of meaning in life.

Spiritual Abuse: When people think of abuse, they don't always consider spiritual or religious institutions. Spiritual abuse occurs when a person forces another to follow their religion or spiritual path. It often involves manipulation and control, usually through fear tactics and harmful beliefs. The most common victims of spiritual abuse are children who are not given the right to think or believe things that are different from the adults around them. They are forced to adhere to tradition against their will and are not allowed to voice their opinions or beliefs. If they have a spiritual experience that does not match their parents' belief system, they are often subjected to contempt, anger, and punishment. However, spiritual abuse can happen to anyone at any age.

Invalidation of Beliefs: Whether spiritual or intellectual, when someone invalidates our beliefs, it invalidates our core identity. The way we view and experience the world is what makes us unique. Our backgrounds and upbringings develop our belief systems and ideas, which give us a unique perspective and help us stand out from others. When someone else invalidates our beliefs, it robs us of our uniqueness. Though not everyone will always agree with us or see things the way we do, we all deserve to be respected for our ideas.

SIGNS OF AN IMBALANCED CROWN CHAKRA

As you may have guessed, an imbalanced crown chakra will often cause problems related to the head and brain. While there are physical ailments that can be influenced by crown chakra blockages, I find the primary concerns are those involving mental health. The crown chakra connects with the mind and soul, and when those are out of balance, we experience severe emotional and mental health challenges. Below is a list of common signs of an imbalanced crown chakra.

Emotional and mental health concerns of the crown chakra include:

- Overintellectualization
- Developmental and learning disabilities
- Anxiety
- Apathy
- Addictions
- Depression
- Psychosis
- Dissociation
- Feeling overwhelmed

Physical ailments tied to the crown chakra include:

- Headaches and migraines
- Brain tumors
- Brain injuries
- Amnesia
- Poor coordination
- Cognitive problems

Life challenges that manifest from an imbalanced crown chakra include:

- Lack of spiritual life/spiritual cynicism
- Learning difficulties
- Spiritual addiction
- Confusion
- Difficulty concentrating
- A need to always be right
- Belief in limitations
- Harmful or severely limiting belief systems

THE CROWN CHAKRA AND THE SHADOW

The Shadow of the crown chakra reveals our toxic thoughts and harmful spiritual habits. If we have any negative relationship involving spirituality, it will be exposed through our Shadow. This can happen in two ways: either your spirituality is diminished, and you aren't connecting with your soul, or you're becoming too obsessed with your spiritual path and ignoring your earthly responsibilities. Let's explore how these manifest.

Spiritual Escapism/Addiction: We did not incarnate on this planet just to run away from all earthly matters. Spirituality is important, but it is not more important than tending to our human life. When many seekers begin their spiritual path, they become hooked on the bliss and joy that comes with reconnecting with their soul. They feel that enlightenment needs to be a 24/7 journey and that all other matters should be dismissed. But if our purpose was to focus purely on spiritual matters, we would not have any earthly concerns.

When this particular Shadow issue arises, it often makes spirituality a form of escapism or addiction. Some will spirituality as a means to shirk responsibilities or avoid the negative aspects of human life. You may think that more spirituality will help you better integrate your soul, but the fact is it has the opposite effect. Our career, family, responsibilities, and friends are all included in who we are, so ignoring these in order to meditate 24/7 creates further disconnection.

Imposing Belief Systems onto Others: Another primary area that can be affected by the Shadow is our belief systems. We all develop a unique perspective on the world based on our backgrounds and experiences, and our resulting belief systems shape our entire experience. But for some, it is not enough for them alone to have their opinions or perspectives. When insecurity mixes with their beliefs, the Shadow causes them to engage in abuse and manipulation. These people use these tactics to impose their beliefs on others because they think they need everyone around them to share their mindset so they can feel somewhat secure with their own.

We can find evidence of this very thing happening right now. People from certain religions feel the need to control and harm others in the name of their beliefs. Racism, sexism, homophobia and antisemitism are all on the rise because some of those in power believe that some people are not equal to others. They manipulate people into thinking the same way and use the power of the 'mind hive' to discriminate against certain groups.

Interestingly, it seems that most people trying to impose their belief systems onto others tend to have perspectives that are harmful to others. I believe that an imbalanced and shadowed crown chakra is what leads to such harmful belief systems. Since Spirit is of pure love and light, it would never encourage humans to treat each other poorly, which tells me that a blockage is usually to blame, and the Shadow exposes this.

Attachment Issues: If you've read a few spiritual books, you are probably familiar with the idea of non-attachment. Non-attachment is the idea that you should not have an emotional attachment to anyone or anything in the earthly realm. Though you can enjoy your friends and some luxuries, the point is to not let these things be the ultimate source of your happiness.

But some people misunderstand this as not owning things or having any people in their life. That life involves pursuing a spiritual path 24/7 and doing nothing else. Because they are so desperate not to own or be attached to anything, they cut people out of their life, quit their jobs, and sell everything they own. Though a select few can do all this and still have a healthy earthly/spirit balance, this is not the case for most people. If attachment is always bad, we wouldn't be on earth developing relationships and enjoying our physical existence. There would be no point to our existence on this planet. Why would we be here if we weren't supposed to enjoy life? In other words, some attachment is perfectly fine. You just don't want to be overly controlling of others or allow an attachment to determine your happiness and self-worth.

On the other hand, this Shadow issue can also show up as overattachment, especially in people who do not have a spiritual life. Any overdependence on anything, whether money, a belief system, a person, or a thing, is equally unhealthy. Again, some attachment is fine, but an overattachment means that the thing you are attached to will always have control over your emotional well-being. Enjoy your friends and family, and don't feel guilty about having some luxuries. Just remember that they are not the source of your happiness and well-being.

The Need to Be Right: When the Shadow dominates the crown chakra, we can become quite stubborn in our beliefs. The Shadow always exposes insecurities, and nothing good comes from mixing insecurity with a stubborn mindset. We become uncomfortable with the idea of being wrong, so we double down on our ideas and try to force people to see things our way because we can't handle being wrong or being contradicted. We might engage in a number of negative behaviors to convince others we're right, including yelling, skewing facts, or ignoring any reality that contradicts what we believe.

HEALING TOOLS TO UNBLOCK YOUR CROWN CHAKRA

Throughout this book, I've listed crystals, essential oils, and foods that can help heal each chakra. Though these healing tools are helpful for all chakras, since they are spiritual healing tools, they have an extra effect on the crown chakra.

Crystals

The best crystals for the crown chakra have high vibrations that help you connect with the spiritual realms. Look for crystals that deepen your meditation practice and help you connect with Spirit in any form it takes

(God, Allah, angels, etc.) Below are a few crystals that I recommend.

- **Celestite:** A beautiful sky-blue stone that heals your worries and anxieties. It also deepens your meditation practice and helps you connect with your soul.
- **Selenite:** A pure white crystal (often found in the shape of a wand) that encourages truth, integrity, and positivity. It also attunes you to higher energies and expands your consciousness.
- **Amethyst:** A popular purple stone that helps with anxiety, stress, and any other negative emotions that block your crown chakra. It deepens your meditation practices, helps you get in touch with your inner wisdom, expands your consciousness, and opens your connection to Spirit.
- **Lepidolite:** A lovely gemstone that showcases various shades of purple and pink. This is a great gem to grab when struggling with anxiety and needing some help in restoring peace. It also helps you with your cosmic connection, processing your fears, and restoring inner happiness.

- **Lapis Lazuli:** A gorgeous dark stone flecked with gold that helps illuminate the mind and awaken your spiritual power.
- **Clear Quartz:** A clear, white crystal that serves as a master healer. It helps remove all blockages and promotes an open mind and heart. It clears blockages in the crown, opening up all connection to higher realms.
- **Labradorite:** A mystical-looking stone that mimics Aurora Borealis, this gemstone helps you connect with your higher self and provides spiritual protection.
- **Sugilite:** A dark purple and very powerful stone that helps you connect your heart to your head. It also clears up the energy that keeps you stuck in the past and prevents you from forgiving others.
- **Fluorite:** This gem comes in many colors and can help with a variety of issues. It clears the mind to improve focus and thought and can deepen your meditation practice. It can also help clear up any confusion in your life.

Essential Oils

When choosing an essential oil for your crown chakra, select those that help you get in touch with the spiritual realms and your soul. Though any of your favorite oils can help you with this (depending on your preferences), here is a list of some essential oils that I recommend.

- Lavender
- Jasmine
- Rose
- Sandalwood
- Vetiver
- Neroli
- Frankincense
- Cedarwood
- Myrrh
- Spikenard

Diet

As with the other chakras, there are some recommended foods that can help stimulate energy in your crown chakra. Essentially, you want to consume white or purple foods and seasonings, as these are the two colors associated with this chakra. Below are a few foods you might wish to incorporate into your diet:

- Coconut
- Garlic
- Ginger
- Onion
- Mushrooms

- Blackberries

That said, diet recommendations for the crown chakra are a bit unique. While other chakras can be healed by specific foods, the general consensus with the crown chakra is that the opposite works. If you want a boost to your crown chakra, fasting is highly recommended. Experts say that spending a few days only consuming purified water, fresh air, and sunshine helps clear any toxins and energies that are blocking you from your full connection to Spirit. However, I always recommend talking with your doctor first to ensure that a fast is a safe option for you.

Meditation

Meditation is the ultimate healing tool for the crown chakra. Though it can help other chakras as well, since it is a form of spiritual communication, it has the strongest effect on the crown chakra. Though there are many forms of meditation, there is not one that is better than the others. As long as you are connecting with your soul and Spirit, your meditation practice can heal your crown chakra.

EXERCISES FOR HEALING THE CROWN CHAKRA

When conducting Shadow work for the crown chakra, focus on exercises that help you create a positive and balanced spiritual life. If you wish to deepen your connection with your soul, the following exercises can help. However, if you are struggling with excessive energy in the crown chakra, I recommend also incorporating the root chakra exercises from Chapter Three to keep yourself grounded.

Journal Prompts

When journaling for the crown chakra, take some time to explore your connection with your soul, spirituality, and the higher powers. Do you have a relationship with these? If not, why not? Below are a few prompts that will help you start exploring these issues.

- Do I feel supported by a higher power? How can I feel more supported and connected?
- Do I feel a calling in my soul? What is this calling?
- Do I believe that I have a life's purpose? What is it? Am I actively working towards it?

- Do I incorporate a spiritual ritual into my daily routine? If not, what spiritual practices can I incorporate?
- What can I do to feel more inner peace?
- When do I impose my beliefs or ideas on others? What can I do to be more open-minded?
- Who is God to me? What can I do to connect to this higher power?
- What can I do to practice spiritual surrender?
- What does spiritual enlightenment mean to me?
- What does my highest, most authentic self look like?

Affirmations

Affirmations can be particularly powerful for opening the crown chakra. They can help you to connect with the divine and bring peace and wisdom to your soul. Below are a few affirmations that can get you started.

- I am guided by my inner wisdom.
- I am open to new ideas.
- The world is my teacher.
- I am connected to the Universe.
- I release all unhealthy attachments.
- I surrender myself to what is.
- I am connected to everyone and everything.

- Spirit runs through me and everything around me.
- Everything is connected.
- Enlightenment is available to me.
- I am grounded and connected.
- I am connected to love and light.
- I am a divine being.
- My connection to Spirit is a priority to me.
- I am my highest, most authentic self.
- I release fear and doubt and welcome faith.
- I am worthy of divine love.
- I know inner peace.
- I am a pure spiritual being.
- I am love. I am light. I am connected to all.

Yoga

Similar to the third eye chakra, you want to incorporate yoga poses that target your head to clear the crown chakra. Below are a few poses that can help.

Sirsasana (Headstand): As the name suggests, this is a headstand and requires great strength and balance to achieve. Begin in a kneeling position and bend forward. Fold your arms into a triangle and place the crown of your head between your interlocked fingers. Lift your legs and walk them towards your head. Bend your knees and lift off. Once your legs are in the air, straighten them upward.

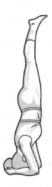

Uttanasana (Standing Forward Fold Pose): From a standing position, slowly bend forward until your head touches your legs. You can either place your fingertips on the ground or wrap your arms around your legs for support.

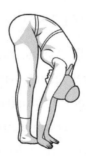

Padmasana (Lotus Pose): Simply sit comfortably on your mat, cross your legs, and place a foot on each thigh. Relax into a deep meditation.

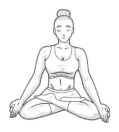

Makarasana (Crocodile Pose): Lie down on your stomach and fold your arms in front of you, resting your head on your arms. This is an easy pose when needing to relax and release any tension.

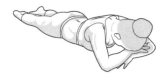

Sarvangasana (Rabbit Stand): From a kneeling position, reach your arms back and grab your heels. Bend forward, letting the crown of your head touch the floor.

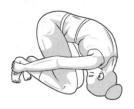

VISUALIZATION MEDITATION

As always, find a comfortable spot to sit or lie down. When opening the crown chakra, it's more important than ever to keep yourself grounded, so be sure to take a few minutes to breathe calmly, deeply, and slowly. Allow each breath to bring you greater awareness of the present moment. Breathe out all tension and allow your mind to settle. Take notice of your surroundings—how the floor feels beneath you, the smells of your home, or even any draft or breeze you feel. Allow yourself to be fully grounded in the moment.

When relaxed and grounded, bring your awareness to a thousand-petalled lotus above your head. This is your crown chakra, the seat of all spiritual communication. It is ready to open up for greater wisdom and spiritual connection. Notice the brilliant light that shines from it. Let this light flow from your crown chakra and spiral down your body.

As you allow the light to move down your body, feel free to speak affirmations to further open up your connection with Spirit. For example, you might say, "I am light," "I am love," or "I am fully connected to the Universe." Say or visualize anything that further improves this connection.

As the light fills your body, do you notice any messages arising? Is Spirit trying to tell you something? Or perhaps you feel some sensations. Maybe a tingling on the top of your head or energy pulsing through your body? Keep breathing deeply and allow these sensations to pass.

Continue this meditation as long as you need. You may be invited to have a conversation with Spirit. If so, take time to converse. When you are finished, allow the light to contract back to the lotus. Thank it for its healing and help. Finally, take a few more deep breaths and slowly open your eyes.

10

INTEGRATION

The majority of this book has been dedicated to exploring each individual chakra in-depth, discussing their themes, what they affect, and how the Shadow manifests in each of them. But it is rare to experience energy blockages that are so obvious or straightforward. The truth is that many of the challenges, hurts, and other adverse situations we encounter in life block more than just one chakra at a time. As for the Shadow, it is a complex archetype that contains a blend of various hurts and beliefs we've picked up over time. Because of this, it is common for people to have multiple imbalanced chakras and a Shadow that requires healing from multiple angles.

In this chapter, I will take a step back and examine the whole picture of chakra and Shadow healing. First, we'll discuss factors that commonly block and imbalance multiple chakras. Then, I'll provide some exercises that help with more general energy and Shadow healing.

COMMON FACTORS THAT NEGATIVELY AFFECT ALL CHAKRAS

If you've read each chapter up until this point, you've probably already noticed that there are recurrent factors that contribute to energy blockages. That's because there are some situations that are so challenging and painful that they affect multiple areas of our lives. Let's revisit these factors but explore their overall effects on our chakras and energy.

Abuse: Abuse is a terrible thing that can completely alter and/or destroy the mental health of the victim. When in an abusive situation, whether it be physical, emotional, or some other form, you lose your sense of safety, identity, and self-worth. Victims often shut down their minds and energy to protect themselves and find themselves completely losing control of their lives. Abusers find ways to manipulate their victims into believing they deserve the abuse, which completely erodes the victim's self-trust, self-love, and self-acceptance. This has devastating effects on every aspect of their life. Depending on the severity and specifics of the abuse, every single chakra can be affected.

Trauma: No one makes it through life without experiencing some sort of major challenge or traumatizing event. While abuse is obviously traumatic, trauma can include many other experiences, such as a death, witnessing a tragedy, or being in any situation where you feel unsafe. Though some people heal from trauma quickly, others become mentally stuck and struggle to move forward with their lives. This can create inertia in multiple areas of one's life, depending on the traumatic event. This can cause imbalances in issues related to survival, communication, self-worth, self-love, and inner or physical vision.

Shame: Shame is one of the most negative emotions that anyone can feel. It is the emotional manifestation of self-rejection. When we feel shame, we wish we did not have a certain trait or feature or that we hadn't done a certain thing. Shame can arise from being overly criticized, experiencing trauma, or feeling embarrassed about an aspect of yourself. It can also arise from guilt or other negative emotions. Sometimes shame is brought upon us through other people's actions, and sometimes our own. Regardless of its origins, feeling shame for any aspect of yourself will cause a significant block in your energy that is bound to affect multiple chakras.

Low Self-Worth: Although the solar plexus is the primary chakra of self-esteem and self-worth, possessing little of each affects other chakras. For example, if you have low self-esteem, you may not feel confident in your creativity or sexuality (sacral chakra issues), or you may not have the courage to speak your inner truth (a throat chakra issue). Low self-worth is often caused by the other factors previously mentioned but in itself can cause severe energetic blockages.

If you have experienced any of these concerns, you probably noticed that many or all of your chakras were blocked or imbalanced while working through this book. As we've discussed, these concerns have deep roots in your energetic system, so it makes sense they would affect multiple chakras. They are also usually at the core of your Shadow work, as many of your limiting beliefs, insecurities, and flaws are directly affected by traumatic events, criticism, and low self-worth.

I find that people who have experienced these issues (especially trauma and abuse) have more work in store for them because instead of healing only one or two areas of their lives, their whole foundation and world have been harmed by these factors. They must work more to build themselves up and restore their natural energetic flow.

This is an important point to understand that most chakra books and blogs don't discuss. If your healing journey is long and complex, it doesn't mean anything is wrong with you or that you are not healing correctly. It may simply mean that you've had a more challenging life than others. But even though the road may seem long and arduous, I'm confident this healing can be done. Below are a few exercises that can help you.

EXERCISES FOR GENERAL HEALING AND INTEGRATION

If you can identify specific chakras that are blocked, then the healing path feels more straightforward. For many, it's not that easy, but this doesn't mean you can't start healing anyway. The rest of this chapter is dedicated to exercises that will help with more general Shadow work and chakra healing. So if you don't know where to start or just want more general healing, then begin with these exercises.

Journal Prompts That Heal the Shadow as a Whole

The following journal prompts will help you pinpoint exactly what areas of your life need healing. By working through these questions, you'll explore what caused you so much pain and how you cope with it. These prompts should also help you find better coping mechanisms and identify specific strategies to further your healing.

- What situation, person, or challenge am I ready to release?
- How does holding onto these painful memories, thoughts, or energy impact my daily life?
- What lessons can I learn from my past?
- How do I cope with my negative thoughts and emotions? Is this healthy?
- How do I react when people trigger my negative emotions?
- What are my emotional triggers? Why do they affect me so much?
- What are some aspects of myself that I don't like? How can I show more love to those parts of myself?
- What memories bring me shame?
- What actions do I deeply regret? Is there any way I can mend the damage?
- What emotions and situations bring out the worst in me?
- What traits or actions do I tend to judge others for? Why am I so judgmental of these things?

- How do I handle anger? What can I do to cope with anger better?
- What are some ways that I can be more loving and kind to the people around me?
- Was there a time in childhood when I felt wronged or abandoned? How does this affect me today?
- Do I have a need to control others? How do I try to bend others to my will?
- What are some instances when I let someone down? Can I mend this?
- Is there anyone whom I have not fully forgiven? Why? Is there any way I can forgive them now?
- What are my boundaries? How can I get better at enforcing them?
- What is the biggest lie I tell myself? Why do I believe it?
- Do I have any toxic traits? How can I heal them into traits that are more positive?

Affirmations for General Shadow Work Healing

Hopefully, by now, you have realized that affirmations are incredibly powerful healing tools. Though people typically use them to heal specific issues, it sometimes helps to use more generic healing statements just to get the process going.

Below are some statements that can help you start your healing journey.

- I choose to move forward and heal.
- I am healing from my past.
- My mistakes do not define me.
- I love all aspects of who I am.
- I love the person I am becoming.
- I forgive myself for all my mistakes.
- I choose to release all grudges and forgive everyone.
- I accept my parents for who they are.
- I accept responsibility for my mistakes.
- My trauma is not my fault.
- I am learning from my past challenges and creating a better future.
- I am not responsible for what happened to me as a child, but I am responsible for how I handle it as an adult.
- The only approval and respect I need is my own.
- My trauma is not an excuse for hurting others; I choose to strive to be better.
- I deserve relationships and situations that lift me up, not ones that drain me.
- I accept that I made mistakes in the past and strive to do better in the future.

- I choose forgiveness because it brings me peace.
- I am growing and healing from my past; I am better than I used to be.
- Facing my emotions makes me stronger.
- I am grateful for every part of me.

YOGA ROUTINES THAT HELP ALL CHAKRAS

Yoga is an incredible activity that helps to keep energy flowing and eliminate blockages. Most yoga poses target one or more chakras, making them an important tool for healing. I've developed two routines that incorporate poses that help each chakra. The first routine is for people who prefer sitting and lying poses. The second routine incorporates more standing poses.

Routine 1

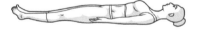

Savasana (Corpse Pose): This is a simple grounding pose. Lie down comfortably on your floor or mat and allow the Earth to support you.

Jathara Parivartanasana (Abdominal Twist): Once you feel supported and grounded, bring your knees to your chest and shift them to one side while keeping your shoulders flat. After a minute or so, twist to the other side.

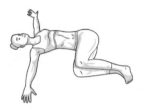

Purvottanasana (Reverse Plank): Sit on the floor with your legs extended in front of you. Prop yourself up on your hands or forearms behind you and raise your hips and abdomen, keeping your palms firmly on the floor. Look up to the ceiling and straighten your body to strengthen your core.

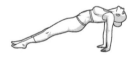

Bhujangasana (Cobra Pose): Lie down on your stomach and with your palms firmly on the ground, lift up your chest and torso. Look to the ceiling and open your chest to fully open the heart.

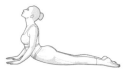

Ustrasana (Camel Pose): Sit on your knees and lean all the way back until your neck is facing the ceiling. Grab your feet to finalize this pose.

Balasana (Child's Pose): Sit on your heels and lean forward, resting your head on the ground. Rest your arms beside your legs, palms out. For a greater stretch in the hips, move your legs further apart. You can also extend your arms out in front of you.

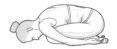

Padmasana (Lotus Pose): Relax your body in a crossed-legged sitting position. Take this time to meditate and reflect on how your energy feels and where you are in life. Sit here as long as you wish and enjoy your meditation.

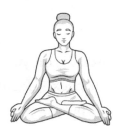

Routine 2

Tadasana (Mountain Pose): Stand straight and tall, with your hands at your sides and palms facing forward. This grounding pose helps energy flow to the root chakra and keeps you rooted to the Earth. For further grounding, you can visualize roots connecting from your feet to the Earth.

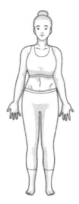

Utkata Konasana (Goddess Pose): From a standing position, move your legs apart and turn your feet outward to either side. Now bend your knees. Lift up your arms and bend them at a 90 degree angle.

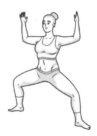

Virabhadrasana II (Warrior II): Stand with your legs shoulder-width apart and your feet firmly planted on the ground. The front foot should face forward while the other faces the side. Extend the front leg into a lunge and lift your arms out to the sides for a powerful, strengthening stance.

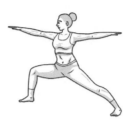

Anjaneyasana (Low Lunge): From Warrior II, relax your arms and deepen your lunge, so the back leg is lowered to the floor. Straighten your arms and lift them up to the sky. Lift up your chest and torso as much as possible to open up your heart and chest.

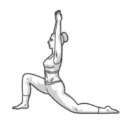

Bhujangasana (Cobra Pose): Lie flat on your stomach and raise your upper body slowly, so your torso is off the ground. Try to stretch through this pose as much as possible as you look towards the ceiling.

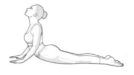

Adho Mukha Svanasana (Downward Facing Dog):
From Cobra Pose, relax your torso and neck, then push
your abdomen and legs up and position yourself into an
upside-down V. Relax your head between your arms or
rest it all the way on the ground if you have the flexibility to do so.

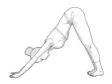

Padmasana (Lotus Pose): Relax your body into a
crossed-legged sitting position. As with the last routine,
take this time to sit in silence and reflect on your
energy flow and life.

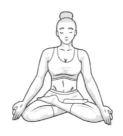

VISUALIZATIONS AND MEDITATIONS

Visualizations are powerful healing techniques. What is happening in your mind's eye is happening for real in the spiritual realm. This means that when you visualize your chakras unblocking, this is actually occurring. This is why it was important for me to add these exercises at the end of each chapter.

For general healing, I offer three more visualization meditations. They will help you unblock your chakras, get grounded, and shield your newly healed energy.

Chakra Meditation

A great way to heal all of your chakras is to have a full visualization session in which you visualize each one. Below is the exercise from Chapter Two to help you with your overall healing journey.

Find a quiet area for your visualization and sit or lie down in a comfortable position. Begin by breathing deeply and slowly and get into a relaxed state.

Now visualize a bright red center at the bottom of your spine. Feel the warmth and energy in that area of your body. This is your root chakra, also known as Muladhara. Imagine it swirling freely and glowing brightly. Let this energy ground you to the Earth and protect you. Feel free to speak some affirmations, such as "I am grounded" or "I am safe."

Move on to your navel, wherein lies the sacral chakra, or Svadhisthana. Visualize the beautiful shade of orange and how it illuminates your whole navel area. Imagine it flowing freely without blockages or stagnation. Do you feel your sexual energy coming alive? Or perhaps your creative energy? Take some time to breathe through any emotions you feel or to repeat affirmations like "I am creative" or "I am sensual."

Repeat this process for all other chakras. Visualize the solar plexus at the top of your stomach, your heart chakra in your chest, your throat chakra in your throat, your third eye on your brow, and the crown chakra on top of your head. Imagine their bright color and their energy flowing freely. Continue to breathe deeply as all that stagnant energy is released. Feel free to recite any affirmations that come to mind during the process.

Once you have gone through each chakra, continue to breathe deeply. Visualize all seven chakras now, all spinning brightly. Notice how good your energy feels. Take a few minutes to enjoy this and get in tune with your energy body. When you are ready, take a few deep breaths and then slowly open your eyes.

Grounding Meditation

When doing any healing work, it is essential to ground yourself so you don't get carried away by the emotions and memories that come with integration. Grounding also keeps you steady so you can more easily navigate life's challenges without being energetically knocked off course. Below is a simple grounding meditation that can keep you rooted throughout all of your challenges.

Find a quiet area for your visualization and stand, sit, or lie down in a comfortable position. Begin by breathing deeply and slowly and get into a relaxed state.

Now, whether standing, sitting, or lying down, take notice of where your body touches the floor. What does the surface feel like? Is it a welcoming feeling? Take note of any other sensations you experience. How do your clothes feel on your skin? What does the temperature feel like? Can you feel a breeze or a draft? Pay attention to anything you feel or experience that keeps you grounded in this moment.

Now notice how the Earth is supporting you, how it holds you up as you do this meditation. Notice how strong and sturdy the Earth is in its foundation and support. It is always here to support you, to help you when everything else becomes unstable.

Now visualize roots extending from your body and winding their way into the ground. These roots are helping you remain grounded so that no matter how far you fly, you will continue to be rooted. These roots go deep into the Earth, helping you feel sturdy when the winds of change and chaos blow. Notice how safe and calm you feel knowing that the Earth will always be here to support you.

Spend as much time as you like connecting with the Earth. When you are finished, express your gratitude for the Earth's support and love. Then slowly open your eyes.

Shielding Meditation

Once you begin healing, be careful to protect your energy so it doesn't become blocked or polluted again. It is crucial to create a shielding routine before you go out and start your day. You can find a shielding charm or crystal, but I've also provided a shielding meditation that will do the trick.

Find a quiet area for your visualization and sit or lie down in a comfortable position. Begin by breathing deeply and slowly and get into a relaxed state.

Now visualize a bright white light descending from heaven to you. This light is warm and comforting; it has arrived to protect you from all harm. Allow the light to shine over you and protect your aura.

Notice how the white light is encompassing you, almost like a large white bubble to keep you shielded. It is a strong and bright shield that deflects anything that is not intended for your benefit. It will protect you from all darkness and harmful energies. Feel its protection as it envelops you.

Allow yourself to sit in this protective shield as long as you like. It will not go away when this meditation ends. However, you should do this visualization often to strengthen it. When you are finished, you can slowly open your eyes.

You don't have to do these three visualization meditations separately. If you wish, you can combine them all into one longer meditation session. But no matter what healing modality you choose, putting in any effort is bound to bring you the relief and peace you crave.

CONCLUSION

Integrating the Shadow is one of the most critical healing journeys anyone can take. It involves tremendous self-awareness and an enormous amount of self-love in order to be successful. To fully integrate our whole psyche, we need to understand our weaknesses, limiting beliefs, and flaws. To succeed in healing, we must love and forgive ourselves and accept our imperfect natures. It is an arduous journey where only the bravest and humblest succeed.

But since you've read this book, I believe in your success. Knowing you need to heal is the first step on your journey. All you have to do now is to commit. Most people fail on their healing journeys because they don't want to face their Shadow. Even if they have the awareness, the pain and shame are too much, so they continue to perpetuate the status quo. But people who do this never change their behaviors, and as a result don't experience relief from their emotional pain, or change their lives. Without facing our Shadow, we can never truly be the person we want to be or live the life of our dreams. Ignoring the Shadow leads to inertia, but integration brings momentum.

And the truth is, ignoring the Shadow is just painful. Though it seems easier to ignore your limiting thoughts, shortcomings, and emotional pain, this can cause more problems than it solves. Not only will you continue to live in distress, but the Shadow will arise in other forms to be noticed, and some of those forms could hurt others around you.

This book has armed you with considerable knowledge and practices that will help you on your journey. As I've explained throughout, healing the chakras is integral to Shadow integration, as each chakra governs some aspect of it. Healing this rainbow bridge one by one is a great way to peer deeper into the Shadow and slowly integrate into wholeness.

A word of caution, though. Just because you have finished this book doesn't mean you're finished with your healing journey. In fact, it's likely that you have only just started. For example, as you did the exercises, did you initially feel great but notice your Shadow issues arise again soon afterward? This is normal, of course, because issues with the Shadow and chakras are often deep and complex, and healing them is a process. Rarely will a Shadow quality be healed after one exercise or session. Naturally, life would be easier if we could simply do one healing session, but unfortunately, life is far more complicated than that. Our traumas and burdens can be quite stubborn and affect multiple areas of our lives, which means you may find your healing journey to be a long one.

But if you find the information and exercises in this book helpful, keep going. Shadow work and chakra healing are ongoing processes that you may work on for years or even throughout your life. Not only are some issues complex and need healing from multiple angles, but people often find that healing one issue reveals other issues that were hidden before.

Furthermore, as you grow older, whether you want it to or not, your Shadow will continue to grow with you. Events will occur that will trigger your Shadow and show you what aspects still need healing. Other situations will cause new pains that will also need to be healed. Though this can be discouraging, I encourage you to keep at it. The more you heal, the better you will feel.

I want to thank you for reading this book and incorporating these exercises and ideas into your healing journey. I know there are numerous books about chakras and healing, so I appreciate that you took the time to read this one.

I also want to thank you for doing this difficult healing work. Not only does working on your Shadow heal you, but it benefits others as well. Integrating your Shadow and healing your chakras encourages you to be more loving and kind, which can only benefit everyone around you. Your joy and love make the world a better place. Healing your Shadow also helps to heal the collective Shadow. The more people work to heal themselves, the more the world heals and becomes a better place to live.

Whatever challenges you face or emotional burdens you carry, I know you can succeed at healing them. Integrating your Shadow is not easy. In fact, I believe it is one of the most challenging things we do on our spiritual path. But I know that healing is possible and that you can experience it yourself. So keep healing, friend, and know that someday you will emerge as a wholly integrated soul.

Made in United States
Troutdale, OR
06/09/2023